# INDEX

**Puzzles** 2-101

**Solutions** 102-126

# #1

| | | | | | | | | |
|---|---|---|---|---|---|---|---|---|
| | | 6 | | | 5 | | | |
| | | | 2 | 1 | | | | 5 |
| 2 | | | | | 4 | | | |
| | 4 | 5 | 6 | | 1 | 2 | 9 | |
| | | | 9 | 3 | | | 4 | |
| 3 | | 7 | | | | | | |
| | 7 | | | | 9 | 3 | 1 | |
| | 2 | | | | | | | |
| | | 1 | | 6 | | | 8 | |

**Solution on page 102**

# #2

| | | | | | | | | |
|---|---|---|---|---|---|---|---|---|
| | | | 3 | | | | | |
| | 5 | 3 | 6 | 8 | | 4 | | 9 |
| 9 | | | | 1 | | | | |
| | 8 | | 1 | 5 | | | | 2 |
| | | 2 | | | 6 | | | 1 |
| 1 | | | | | 3 | | | 5 |
| | | | | 9 | | | 7 | |
| 6 | | | | | | 2 | | |
| | 1 | | | | | | 5 | 4 |

**Solution on page 102**

# #3

| | | | | | | | | |
|---|---|---|---|---|---|---|---|---|
| 8 | 5 | 6 | 3 | | | | | 4 |
| | | | 4 | 6 | | | | |
| | 9 | | 5 | | | 7 | | |
| 6 | | | 8 | 1 | | | | |
| | | | | | | | 7 | |
| | | | | | 4 | 6 | | 8 |
| | 6 | 9 | | | 5 | | 1 | |
| | 2 | 4 | 1 | | | | | 7 |
| | | 1 | | 2 | | 3 | | |

**Solution on page 102**

# #4

| | | | | | | | | |
|---|---|---|---|---|---|---|---|---|
| | | 2 | 3 | | | | | |
| 3 | | | | | 9 | 4 | | |
| | | | | 5 | | 6 | 9 | |
| 8 | | | | | 2 | 9 | | 6 |
| | | 4 | | 3 | | 7 | | |
| | | 3 | 1 | | | | 4 | 8 |
| 2 | | | | 9 | 7 | | | 5 |
| | | | | | | | | |
| | 1 | 6 | | | | 8 | | |

**Solution on page 102**

# #5

| | | | | | | | | |
|---|---|---|---|---|---|---|---|---|
| | | | | | 5 | | | |
| | | | 1 | | | 4 | | |
| | | 8 | | 3 | | | | 1 |
| | 6 | | | | | 1 | | |
| | 5 | | | | | | 7 | |
| 4 | | 9 | 6 | 1 | | | 5 | |
| | | 5 | | 2 | 1 | | | 9 |
| | 7 | | | 4 | | | 2 | |
| | 2 | | | 9 | | 7 | | 3 |

**Solution on page 103**

# #6

| | | | | | | | | |
|---|---|---|---|---|---|---|---|---|
| 7 | | 6 | | 2 | 1 | | | |
| | | | | | 6 | | 1 | 4 |
| | | 9 | | | | | | |
| 8 | | 5 | | | | | 2 | |
| | | | | | 5 | | 7 | 1 |
| | | | 1 | | | | 6 | |
| | | 1 | 6 | | 9 | | | 3 |
| | | | 4 | | 3 | 9 | 8 | 7 |
| 9 | | 8 | | | | | | |

**Solution on page 103**

# #7

| | | | | | | | | |
|---|---|---|---|---|---|---|---|---|
| | | | 5 | 9 | | | | 2 |
| | 9 | | | | | | | |
| 7 | 3 | 1 | 2 | | | 9 | | |
| | | 8 | 1 | | 7 | | | |
| | 4 | | | | 8 | 2 | | 7 |
| | 1 | 7 | | | | 3 | 9 | |
| | | 6 | 8 | | | 4 | | |
| | | | | | 6 | 8 | 7 | |
| | | 3 | | 4 | | | | |

**Solution on page 103**

# #8

| | | | | | | | | |
|---|---|---|---|---|---|---|---|---|
| 5 | 3 | | 2 | 6 | | 1 | | |
| | | 7 | | | 3 | | | |
| 1 | | | | | | | | 2 |
| | | | 6 | | 5 | 3 | | 4 |
| | | | 3 | | | | 9 | 7 |
| 6 | | | 1 | 4 | | | | |
| | | | | | | | | |
| | | | 8 | | 9 | 7 | | 1 |
| 2 | | | | | | | 5 | 3 |

**Solution on page 103**

# #9

| | | | | | | | | |
|---|---|---|---|---|---|---|---|---|
| 3 | 4 | | | | | | | |
| 7 | | | | | 6 | | | 8 |
| | 1 | | 7 | 5 | | 3 | 2 | |
| 6 | 9 | | | 7 | | | | |
| | | 3 | 5 | | | | 8 | |
| | | 4 | 2 | | | 7 | | 9 |
| | | | | 8 | | | | |
| | | | 6 | | 9 | 2 | | |
| | 5 | 1 | | | | | | |

**Solution on page 104**

# #10

| | | | | | | | | |
|---|---|---|---|---|---|---|---|---|
| | 7 | 9 | | | | 4 | 1 | 3 |
| | 3 | | | 9 | | | 6 | |
| | | | | | 1 | | | |
| | | | | 4 | 2 | | | |
| 4 | | | | 6 | | | 7 | 5 |
| | | 6 | | 3 | | 9 | | |
| | | 1 | | | | | | |
| 9 | | | 8 | | | | | 4 |
| | | 5 | 7 | | 6 | 2 | | |

**Solution on page 104**

# #11

| | | | | | | | | |
|---|---|---|---|---|---|---|---|---|
| 4 | | 8 | | 5 | | | | |
| | | | | | | 6 | 9 | |
| | | | | | 7 | | | |
| | | 3 | | 9 | 2 | 4 | 1 | 6 |
| 9 | | | 4 | | | 8 | | |
| | | 1 | 5 | | | | 3 | |
| | | 7 | | 2 | 5 | | 6 | |
| 6 | | | 7 | | | | | |
| 1 | | | | | 9 | | 7 | |

**Solution on page 104**

# #12

| | | | | | | | | |
|---|---|---|---|---|---|---|---|---|
| 8 | | | | | | 1 | | 7 |
| | 2 | 6 | 8 | | 7 | | 5 | |
| | | 3 | | | | | 8 | |
| | | | | | | | 1 | 3 |
| 6 | | | | 8 | | | 4 | 2 |
| 4 | | | 1 | | | 7 | | |
| | | 5 | | | 4 | | | 8 |
| | | 4 | | | | 3 | | |
| 7 | | | | | 8 | | 2 | |

**Solution on page 104**

# #13

| | | | | | | | | |
|---|---|---|---|---|---|---|---|---|
| 4 | 6 | | 3 | | | | | |
| | | | | 4 | | | | |
| | 2 | 3 | | 8 | 6 | | | |
| | 4 | 2 | 1 | 5 | | | 3 | 6 |
| | | 9 | | | | | 8 | 4 |
| | | | 2 | | | | 5 | |
| | 3 | 7 | | | | | | 2 |
| | | | 9 | | | | | |
| | | | | | 5 | 7 | | |

**Solution on page 105**

# #14

| | | | | | | | | |
|---|---|---|---|---|---|---|---|---|
| 8 | | | | | 7 | 9 | 3 | |
| 9 | | | 1 | 8 | | 6 | | |
| | | 2 | | | 4 | | | |
| | 1 | | | 6 | | | | |
| | 8 | | | | | 2 | | 4 |
| | | | | 4 | | 3 | 9 | |
| 2 | | | | 9 | | 1 | 7 | |
| | | 3 | | | | | | |
| | | | 2 | | 8 | | | |

Solution on page 105

# #15

| | | | | | | | | |
|---|---|---|---|---|---|---|---|---|
| | | | 5 | | 4 | | | |
| 5 | | 2 | | | | | | 9 |
| 7 | | | 2 | 3 | 9 | | 8 | |
| | | | | | | | 2 | 6 |
| | 5 | 6 | | 7 | | | | |
| 2 | | | | 4 | | 7 | 9 | |
| | 7 | | | 9 | 6 | | | |
| | | 1 | | | | | | 7 |
| | 8 | | | | | | 6 | 3 |

**Solution on page 105**

# #16

| | | | | | | | | |
|---|---|---|---|---|---|---|---|---|
| 4 | | 5 | 9 | | | | | 6 |
| | | | | 4 | | | 2 | |
| | 2 | | 5 | | | 3 | | |
| | | 9 | 7 | | 1 | 2 | 6 | |
| | | 6 | | 9 | | | | |
| 2 | 1 | | 6 | | | | | |
| | 6 | | | 1 | | 7 | | |
| | | | | | 8 | | | 3 |
| 3 | | 2 | | | 5 | 8 | | |

**Solution on page 105**

# #17

|   |   |   |   |   |   |   |   |   |
|---|---|---|---|---|---|---|---|---|
|   |   | 5 |   |   |   |   |   | 3 |
|   |   | 7 |   |   |   |   |   |   |
|   |   |   | 7 | 5 |   | 6 | 2 |   |
|   | 2 |   |   |   | 9 | 5 |   | 6 |
|   | 3 |   | 5 |   |   |   | 7 |   |
| 8 |   | 4 |   |   |   |   | 9 |   |
| 3 |   |   | 9 |   |   |   | 4 | 7 |
|   |   |   |   | 2 | 8 |   | 1 |   |
|   |   | 2 |   | 4 |   |   |   |   |

Solution on page 106

# #18

| | | | | | | | | |
|---|---|---|---|---|---|---|---|---|
| 4 | | | | 1 | | 3 | | 6 |
| | 3 | | | | 8 | | | 4 |
| 9 | | | 4 | | | | | |
| 6 | | | | | 7 | | 8 | |
| | | | | 2 | | | | 9 |
| 8 | | | 5 | 9 | 6 | | | |
| 7 | | | 6 | 5 | | | 4 | |
| | | | | | 4 | 2 | | 3 |
| | | 4 | 1 | | 3 | | 7 | |

**Solution on page 106**

# #19

| | | | | | | | | |
|---|---|---|---|---|---|---|---|---|
| 9 | | | 1 | | | 5 | | |
| 6 | | 3 | | | | 4 | | |
| | | 2 | 7 | | 5 | | | |
| | | | | | | | 3 | 2 |
| | | 7 | | 9 | 1 | 8 | | 5 |
| | | 1 | | 3 | | | 9 | |
| | | | 8 | | | 7 | | |
| | 8 | | | | | | 5 | |
| 2 | | | 3 | 7 | | | | |

**Solution on page 106**

# #20

| | | | | | | | | |
|---|---|---|---|---|---|---|---|---|
| 1 | | | | | | 8 | 9 | |
| | | | 5 | 2 | | | | 4 |
| | | | | | 3 | | | |
| | | | 2 | | | | 1 | |
| 4 | 6 | | | | | | | 9 |
| | | 2 | | 8 | | | 4 | |
| | | 4 | | | | | | |
| | 3 | 7 | 1 | | | 4 | | 8 |
| | | 1 | 8 | 4 | | | 6 | 5 |

Solution on page 106

# #21

| | | | | | | | | |
|---|---|---|---|---|---|---|---|---|
| | | 2 | | | | | | |
| | 9 | | | | | 5 | | 8 |
| 8 | | 5 | 6 | | 2 | | 4 | |
| 2 | 4 | 7 | | | | 9 | | |
| | | 3 | 1 | | | | | 7 |
| | | | | 2 | 9 | | | |
| | 1 | 6 | 9 | | 7 | | | 2 |
| | | | | 4 | | 7 | 3 | 1 |
| | | | | | | | | |

**Solution on page 107**

# #22

| | | | | | | | | |
|---|---|---|---|---|---|---|---|---|
| 8 | 6 | | | 5 | | | | 2 |
| 9 | | | | | | 4 | | |
| | | | | | 7 | | 6 | |
| | | 8 | 6 | | 9 | | 3 | |
| | | 2 | | | | 8 | | |
| 1 | | | | 4 | | 5 | | 7 |
| 6 | 1 | 3 | | | | 9 | | |
| | | | 8 | | | | | |
| 2 | | | | 9 | | | 7 | |

**Solution on page 107**

# #23

| | | | | | | | | |
|---|---|---|---|---|---|---|---|---|
| | | | | | | | 4 | |
| | | | | 7 | 1 | | 2 | |
| 5 | 4 | | 9 | 2 | | | 7 | |
| 1 | | | | | | | | |
| | | 3 | 8 | 6 | | | | |
| | 6 | | 5 | | 2 | | | |
| | 3 | | | | 8 | 9 | | |
| | | 4 | | 9 | | | 3 | |
| 8 | | | 2 | | | | 6 | 1 |

**Solution on page 107**

# #24

|   |   |   |   |   |   |   |   |   |
|---|---|---|---|---|---|---|---|---|
|   |   | 6 |   |   | 4 |   |   |   |
|   |   |   | 3 |   |   | 1 | 8 |   |
| 2 |   | 3 | 1 |   |   | 7 |   |   |
|   |   |   |   | 7 |   |   | 1 | 2 |
|   |   |   |   |   | 6 |   | 4 |   |
| 3 |   |   | 2 |   |   |   |   |   |
| 8 |   |   | 9 |   | 7 |   |   |   |
| 7 |   |   |   |   |   | 2 |   |   |
| 1 | 3 |   |   | 5 | 8 |   | 9 |   |

**Solution on page 107**

# #25

|   |   |   |   |   |   |   |   |   |
|---|---|---|---|---|---|---|---|---|
|   | 2 |   | 3 |   |   |   |   | 7 |
|   |   | 4 | 5 | 7 | 6 | 2 |   |   |
|   |   |   |   | 8 |   | 6 | 5 |   |
| 1 |   |   |   | 4 |   |   |   |   |
|   | 4 |   |   |   | 7 |   |   |   |
|   |   |   |   |   |   | 3 | 8 |   |
| 6 |   |   |   |   |   |   |   |   |
| 4 | 3 |   | 9 | 2 | 1 |   | 7 |   |
| 7 |   |   | 4 |   |   |   |   | 9 |

**Solution on page 108**

# #26

| | | | | | | | | |
|---|---|---|---|---|---|---|---|---|
| | | | | | 8 | | | 1 |
| | 7 | | | | | 4 | | |
| 6 | | | | | | 5 | | 9 |
| 8 | | | | 6 | | 2 | | |
| | 9 | 7 | | 5 | | | 3 | |
| | | | | 4 | | | 1 | 7 |
| | 4 | | 9 | | | | | |
| | | | | | 6 | | | |
| | 5 | 1 | | | | | | 4 |

Solution on page 108

# #27

| | | | | | | | | |
|---|---|---|---|---|---|---|---|---|
| | | | | | 7 | | 8 | |
| 5 | | 2 | | | | 9 | | |
| | 3 | | | | 9 | | 7 | |
| | | 1 | | 3 | | 7 | | |
| | | 7 | | | | | 3 | 5 |
| | | | | | | 1 | | |
| | 2 | | 4 | 9 | | | | |
| 6 | | 8 | 2 | | | | 9 | |
| 9 | | | 1 | | | 8 | 2 | |

**Solution on page 108**

# #28

| | | | | | | | | |
|---|---|---|---|---|---|---|---|---|
| | | | 9 | | 2 | | | |
| | | | | | | | 1 | 7 |
| | 4 | 8 | 6 | | | | | |
| | 6 | 3 | 2 | | 1 | | | |
| 1 | | | | | 7 | | 9 | |
| | | | 3 | | | 5 | | |
| | 7 | | | | | | 2 | |
| 5 | 1 | 4 | | 2 | | | 3 | 6 |
| | | 6 | | | | 8 | | |

**Solution on page 108**

# #29

| | | | | | | | | |
|---|---|---|---|---|---|---|---|---|
| 3 | | | 4 | | | 1 | 2 | |
| 6 | | 2 | | | | | | |
| | | | 9 | | | | 6 | |
| | | | 2 | | 1 | | 4 | 8 |
| | 6 | | | | | | | |
| | 8 | | | | | 3 | | 2 |
| | 5 | | | 2 | 8 | 7 | | 9 |
| | | | 1 | 3 | 9 | | | |
| | | 8 | | | 4 | | 3 | |

**Solution on page 109**

# #30

| | | | | | | | | |
|---|---|---|---|---|---|---|---|---|
| | | 7 | | 2 | | 4 | | |
| 1 | | 6 | | | 5 | | 7 | |
| | | | 3 | | | | | 1 |
| 3 | | | | | 2 | | | 5 |
| 6 | | | | | | 1 | | 9 |
| | 1 | | | 7 | | 6 | | |
| 7 | 8 | | | | | | 9 | |
| | | | | | 8 | | | |
| | | 2 | | 4 | | 3 | | |

**Solution on page 109**

# #31

| | | | | | | | | |
|---|---|---|---|---|---|---|---|---|
| | | | | 1 | | 4 | 2 | |
| 3 | | | | | | | 5 | |
| | | | 8 | 9 | | | | |
| | 7 | 6 | | | 4 | 1 | | |
| | | | | 5 | | 8 | | |
| | | | 1 | | 8 | | | |
| | | 2 | 9 | 8 | | | 4 | |
| 7 | 9 | 3 | 4 | | | | 8 | |
| | 6 | | 3 | | | | | 1 |

**Solution on page 109**

# #32

| | | | | | | | | |
|---|---|---|---|---|---|---|---|---|
| 3 | | | | 1 | 9 | | | 4 |
| | 5 | | | | | 7 | | |
| | | 4 | | | | 5 | | 6 |
| | | 9 | | 7 | 2 | | | |
| 2 | | | | | 4 | | | |
| | 3 | | | | | 4 | | |
| | | 5 | | | 3 | | 7 | |
| | | | 8 | | | 9 | | |
| | | 8 | 4 | | | | 2 | |

**Solution on page 109**

# #33

| | | | | | | | | |
|---|---|---|---|---|---|---|---|---|
| | 5 | | 8 | | | 4 | | 9 |
| | | | 6 | | | | | 8 |
| | | | | | 3 | 5 | | |
| | 3 | 7 | | 9 | | | 1 | |
| | 1 | | 3 | 8 | | 6 | | |
| | 6 | | | | | | 8 | |
| | | 9 | | | 8 | | | |
| | | | 4 | | | | | 1 |
| 6 | | | | | 7 | | 5 | 3 |

**Solution on page 110**

# #34

| | | | | | | | | |
|---|---|---|---|---|---|---|---|---|
| | | 5 | | | | 9 | | |
| 7 | 8 | | | 6 | | | | |
| | | | 8 | 7 | | 4 | | |
| 6 | | 2 | 9 | | | | 3 | |
| | | 4 | 7 | | | | | |
| | | 9 | | 8 | | | | 1 |
| | 4 | | | | | 2 | 7 | 9 |
| | 9 | | | | 1 | | | |
| 3 | | 8 | | | | | | |

**Solution on page 110**

# #35

| | | | | | | | | |
|---|---|---|---|---|---|---|---|---|
| 2 | | | | 1 | | 8 | 5 | 4 |
| | | 6 | | | | | | 9 |
| | | | | | 7 | | | 1 |
| 4 | 2 | | 8 | | | 5 | | |
| 7 | | 9 | | | | | 8 | 2 |
| | | | | 5 | | | 9 | |
| | 6 | | 9 | | 2 | 1 | | 8 |
| | 9 | | 3 | | 1 | | | |

**Solution on page 110**

# #36

| | | | | | | | | |
|---|---|---|---|---|---|---|---|---|
| | | 7 | | 3 | | | | |
| | | | 1 | 5 | | 4 | | 3 |
| | | | | 8 | 2 | | | |
| | | | | | | 3 | | 7 |
| | 4 | | 2 | 6 | 1 | | 5 | |
| 9 | | 2 | | | | | | |
| 3 | | 4 | | | | | 7 | |
| | | | | | | 9 | | 6 |
| | | 1 | | | 9 | | | 4 |

**Solution on page 110**

# #37

| | | | | | | | | |
|---|---|---|---|---|---|---|---|---|
| | | 1 | | 3 | | 4 | | 8 |
| | | 6 | | | 8 | | | |
| 3 | | | | 4 | 6 | | 1 | |
| 1 | | | | | 3 | 5 | | |
| | | | | 1 | | | 2 | |
| 7 | 2 | | | | 5 | 1 | | |
| | | | | 8 | 7 | 6 | 4 | |
| | | | | | | | 9 | 2 |
| 9 | | 7 | | 5 | | | | |

**Solution on page 111**

# #38

| | | | | | | | | |
|---|---|---|---|---|---|---|---|---|
| | | | | 2 | | | | |
| | 3 | 4 | | | | | | 7 |
| | | 8 | 6 | | 3 | | | |
| | 5 | | | | 9 | | | |
| 3 | | 6 | 5 | | | | 8 | 1 |
| | | | | 3 | | 5 | | |
| | 1 | 5 | | 7 | | | | |
| | | | | | | 7 | | 9 |
| | 7 | | 3 | | 1 | | 5 | 2 |

**Solution on page 111**

# #39

| | | | | | | | | |
|---|---|---|---|---|---|---|---|---|
| | 5 | | | | | | | |
| 8 | | 1 | | | | 5 | 7 | |
| | | | | | | 4 | | 3 |
| | | 3 | | 6 | | 7 | | |
| 2 | | | | 8 | 5 | 9 | | |
| | | 9 | | | | | 5 | 6 |
| 6 | | | | 4 | | | 2 | |
| | | | 6 | | | 3 | 8 | |
| | 2 | 7 | | 9 | | | | |

**Solution on page 111**

# #40

| | | | | | | | | |
|---|---|---|---|---|---|---|---|---|
| | | | 1 | 8 | | | | 9 |
| 5 | | | | | | 8 | | 2 |
| | | 8 | | | | 6 | 4 | |
| | | 2 | 6 | 1 | | | | |
| | | 5 | | | | | | |
| | | | 3 | | 2 | 4 | | |
| | 5 | | | | | 7 | 6 | |
| | 8 | 6 | 7 | | | | | |
| 2 | | 7 | | 6 | 3 | | 8 | 5 |

**Solution on page 111**

# #41

| | | | | | | | | |
|---|---|---|---|---|---|---|---|---|
| | | 1 | | | 6 | | | 4 |
| | | 7 | | 8 | | 5 | | |
| | | | 7 | | 9 | 6 | | |
| | | 9 | | 4 | 1 | | | 7 |
| | | | | 2 | | | | |
| | | | | | | 9 | | |
| | 5 | | | 9 | | 4 | 3 | |
| 7 | | | 1 | | | | | 5 |
| | | 3 | 8 | | 4 | | 9 | |

**Solution on page 112**

# #42

| | | | | | | | | |
|---|---|---|---|---|---|---|---|---|
| | | 6 | 8 | | | | | |
| 2 | 5 | | | 4 | | | | |
| 7 | | | | | | | 2 | |
| | | 4 | 1 | | | | | 6 |
| | | | | | 7 | | 4 | 3 |
| | 9 | | 4 | 5 | | 1 | | |
| | | | 7 | | | | | |
| 1 | | 8 | | 2 | 6 | | | 9 |
| 4 | 6 | | | | | | | 2 |

**Solution on page 112**

# #43

| | | | | | | | | |
|---|---|---|---|---|---|---|---|---|
| 8 | 9 | | | | | | 7 | 3 |
| 7 | | | | 6 | | 1 | | |
| | | | | | | | | 5 |
| 9 | | 8 | | | | 6 | | |
| | 4 | | 6 | | 3 | 8 | | |
| | | | 1 | | | | | |
| 2 | | | | | 1 | | | |
| 6 | 8 | 9 | 5 | | | | 1 | |
| 1 | | | | 8 | | | | 7 |

**Solution on page 112**

# #44

| | | | | | | | | |
|---|---|---|---|---|---|---|---|---|
| | | | | 5 | | 1 | | 4 |
| 1 | | | | 4 | | 2 | | 9 |
| | | | 8 | | 2 | | | |
| 7 | 4 | 6 | | | | | | |
| | | | | 2 | | | | 5 |
| | 9 | 5 | | | 1 | 4 | | |
| 6 | | 4 | | 8 | | | | |
| | | | 3 | | | | | 7 |
| 5 | | 8 | | 7 | | | | 1 |

**Solution on page 112**

# #45

| | | | | | | | | |
|---|---|---|---|---|---|---|---|---|
| | 7 | | | | | | 5 | 2 |
| 4 | | | | | | | 7 | |
| 6 | 8 | | | | | | 4 | 1 |
| | | 5 | | 9 | 6 | | | 4 |
| | | 8 | | 3 | | 1 | | |
| | 1 | | | | 2 | | | |
| 1 | | | | | 4 | | | |
| | | | | 6 | | 9 | | 8 |
| | | | | | 5 | | | 3 |

**Solution on page 113**

# #46

| | | | | | | | | |
|---|---|---|---|---|---|---|---|---|
| | | | | | | | 9 | 6 |
| | | | | 6 | 8 | | | |
| | 5 | | 4 | | | 1 | | |
| | | 7 | 1 | 4 | | | | 2 |
| | 9 | | | 7 | | 4 | 5 | |
| | | | | | 2 | | | 7 |
| | | | | | | | 6 | 4 |
| 3 | 2 | | | | | | | |
| 1 | 4 | | 5 | 3 | 6 | | | |

**Solution on page 113**

# #47

| | | | | | | | | |
|---|---|---|---|---|---|---|---|---|
| | | 4 | 9 | | | | 8 | |
| | | | 3 | 7 | | | 5 | |
| | | | 5 | | 2 | | | |
| | 7 | | | | | | | 6 |
| | 6 | | | 8 | | 1 | | 9 |
| 5 | | 1 | 2 | 6 | | 8 | | |
| | | | | | | 7 | | |
| | | 2 | | | | | | |
| | | 8 | | | 1 | | 6 | |

**Solution on page 113**

# #48

| | | | | | | | | |
|---|---|---|---|---|---|---|---|---|
| | | | | 2 | | | | |
| 2 | | | | 8 | | | | 3 |
| | | | 6 | | | 4 | | 8 |
| 5 | | 2 | 4 | | 1 | | | |
| | | 6 | | | 5 | 1 | | |
| 9 | | | 8 | | | | | |
| | | 1 | | | 9 | | 3 | |
| | 9 | | | | | | | 5 |
| | 5 | | | | | 9 | 8 | 7 |

**Solution on page 113**

# #49

|   |   |   |   |   |   |   |   |   |
|---|---|---|---|---|---|---|---|---|
|   |   | 1 |   |   | 8 | 2 |   |   |
| 3 |   | 4 |   |   |   |   | 8 |   |
|   | 8 |   |   | 7 | 4 |   |   |   |
|   | 1 |   |   |   | 9 | 8 |   |   |
|   |   |   |   | 3 | 7 |   | 5 |   |
| 5 |   | 3 | 2 |   |   | 6 | 7 |   |
|   | 7 | 5 |   |   |   |   |   | 8 |
|   |   |   |   |   |   | 7 |   |   |
|   |   | 6 |   |   |   | 9 | 3 |   |

**Solution on page 114**

# #50

| | | | | | | | | |
|---|---|---|---|---|---|---|---|---|
| | 5 | | | | | | 1 | |
| 2 | | | 6 | | | 5 | | |
| | 3 | | | 2 | | | | 7 |
| 8 | | | 9 | | | | | |
| | 7 | | 3 | 6 | | | 5 | 9 |
| | | 2 | | 8 | | | | |
| 9 | | | | | 1 | 4 | | 3 |
| | 1 | | | | 3 | 6 | 9 | |
| | | | 4 | 9 | | | | |

**Solution on page 114**

# #51

| | | | | | | | | |
|---|---|---|---|---|---|---|---|---|
| | | 3 | | 4 | | | | |
| | | 1 | 3 | | 7 | | | |
| 6 | | | | | 1 | | 2 | 8 |
| | 1 | 9 | | 7 | | | 4 | |
| | | | | 5 | 2 | | 8 | |
| 3 | | | | | | 6 | | |
| 9 | | | | | 5 | 8 | 1 | |
| 4 | | | | | | | | |
| | 7 | | | | | | 5 | 4 |

**Solution on page 114**

# #52

| | | | | | | | | |
|---|---|---|---|---|---|---|---|---|
| 8 | 5 | | 1 | 4 | | | | 2 |
| 3 | | | | 2 | | 7 | | |
| | | | | | | | 8 | 9 |
| 7 | 9 | 4 | | | | | | |
| | | | 4 | | | | | |
| 1 | | | | 8 | 7 | 9 | 6 | |
| | | | | | | | 7 | 8 |
| 5 | | | | | | 3 | | |
| | | 3 | 7 | 1 | | | 5 | |

**Solution on page 114**

# #53

|   |   |   |   |   |   |   |   |   |
|---|---|---|---|---|---|---|---|---|
|   | 7 | 1 |   | 2 |   | 4 |   |   |
|   | 6 |   |   |   |   |   |   |   |
|   | 8 |   |   |   |   | 6 | 2 |   |
|   | 5 |   | 2 |   |   |   |   |   |
| 9 |   |   |   |   | 7 | 2 |   | 1 |
| 4 | 2 | 7 | 1 |   |   |   | 8 |   |
|   |   |   |   |   |   | 1 | 5 |   |
| 8 |   |   |   | 5 | 6 |   |   | 2 |
|   |   |   |   |   |   |   | 9 | 8 |

**Solution on page 115**

# #54

| | | | | | | | | |
|---|---|---|---|---|---|---|---|---|
| 6 | 4 | | | 9 | | | | |
| 7 | | | 8 | | | | | 5 |
| | | 9 | | | | | | |
| | | 4 | | | | 7 | 9 | 2 |
| 2 | 1 | 8 | | | | | | 3 |
| | | | | | | 4 | | |
| | 5 | | 2 | | 7 | | 4 | |
| | 6 | | 4 | 5 | | 8 | | |
| | | | | 8 | | | | |

**Solution on page 115**

# #55

| | | | | | | | | |
|---|---|---|---|---|---|---|---|---|
| 8 | | | | | 6 | | 9 | |
| | | | | | | 5 | | 4 |
| | | 5 | 2 | 9 | | 6 | | |
| | | 2 | | 6 | 3 | | | 5 |
| | 8 | | | | | | 3 | |
| | 4 | | 1 | 8 | | | | |
| | | 9 | | | | | | 2 |
| | | | | | 2 | 7 | 1 | |
| | | | 6 | 3 | 9 | | | |

**Solution on page 115**

# #56

| | | | | | | | | |
|---|---|---|---|---|---|---|---|---|
| | | 2 | 9 | | | | | |
| 7 | 5 | | | 6 | 8 | 1 | | |
| | | 1 | | 4 | | | | |
| | 4 | 6 | | | 7 | | 5 | |
| | 3 | | 8 | | | | | 4 |
| 9 | | | | | | | | |
| | 1 | | | | 9 | | 8 | |
| | | 9 | | | | | | |
| | | | 4 | 5 | | | 6 | 2 |

**Solution on page 115**

# #57

| | | | | | | | | |
|---|---|---|---|---|---|---|---|---|
| | 4 | | | | | 9 | | |
| | | | 8 | | 5 | | | 7 |
| | | | 3 | | | 4 | | |
| 2 | | 3 | | 5 | | 1 | | |
| | 1 | | | 3 | | | 4 | |
| | | | | 1 | | | | 8 |
| 4 | | 9 | 6 | | 7 | | | |
| | | | | | | 5 | | |
| 6 | 7 | 1 | | | | | | |

**Solution on page 116**

# #58

| | | | | | | | | |
|---|---|---|---|---|---|---|---|---|
| | | 3 | | | 8 | 2 | 5 | |
| 7 | | | 6 | | 9 | | | |
| | | | 1 | | 2 | | | 9 |
| | | | | | | 1 | | |
| | | 5 | | | | | | |
| | 9 | 2 | | 6 | | 5 | | 8 |
| | | 8 | | | | | | |
| | | | 5 | | 1 | 7 | | 4 |
| | | 6 | 9 | 7 | | | | |

**Solution on page 116**

# #59

| | | | | | | | | |
|---|---|---|---|---|---|---|---|---|
| 8 | | | | | 7 | | 5 | 3 |
| 3 | | | 8 | | | 2 | | |
| | | 6 | | | | | | |
| | | | | 5 | 6 | | 8 | |
| 6 | 1 | | 4 | | | | 7 | |
| 5 | | 9 | 1 | 7 | | | | |
| | | | 3 | | | 4 | | |
| 9 | | | | | | 5 | | 1 |
| | 6 | 1 | | 9 | | | 3 | |

**Solution on page 116**

# #60

| | | | | | | | | |
|---|---|---|---|---|---|---|---|---|
| 8 | | 1 | | | 3 | 7 | | 2 |
| | | | | 2 | 9 | | 8 | |
| | | | 1 | | | 4 | | |
| 6 | 3 | | | | 1 | | 9 | |
| | | 4 | | | | 3 | | 8 |
| | | | 5 | | | 2 | | |
| 5 | | | | 7 | | | 2 | |
| | | | 9 | 8 | | | | 4 |
| | | 6 | | | 2 | | | |

**Solution on page 116**

# #61

| | | | | | | | | |
|---|---|---|---|---|---|---|---|---|
| | | | | 7 | 1 | 4 | | |
| 1 | | 9 | | | | | | 7 |
| | 5 | | | 9 | | | | |
| 7 | | 1 | | 8 | | | | |
| | | | 1 | | | | | 6 |
| | 2 | 8 | | | 5 | | | 4 |
| | 7 | | | | | | 8 | 3 |
| | 1 | | 7 | 2 | | | | |
| | | 2 | 6 | | | | | |

**Solution on page 117**

# #62

|   |   |   |   |   |   |   |   |   |
|---|---|---|---|---|---|---|---|---|
|   | 1 |   |   | 2 | 6 |   |   |   |
| 2 |   |   |   |   | 8 |   | 9 |   |
|   |   |   | 4 | 9 | 3 |   |   | 2 |
| 6 |   | 7 |   |   |   | 8 |   |   |
|   | 4 |   |   | 8 | 7 | 5 | 1 |   |
|   |   | 8 |   |   |   |   |   |   |
|   |   | 1 | 8 | 4 |   |   |   |   |
|   |   |   |   | 6 | 9 |   |   |   |
| 9 |   |   |   |   | 5 |   | 4 | 7 |

**Solution on page 117**

# #63

| | | | | | | | | |
|---|---|---|---|---|---|---|---|---|
| | | | | | | | | |
| | 3 | | | | 9 | | 1 | 8 |
| 7 | 4 | | | | | 6 | 3 | 9 |
| | 8 | | | 4 | | | | |
| 3 | 6 | | | 2 | 7 | 4 | | 1 |
| | | | | | 6 | | | |
| | | | | | | | | |
| 2 | 7 | | 6 | | 1 | | 9 | 3 |
| | 1 | | 9 | | 3 | 2 | | |

**Solution on page 117**

# #64

| | | | | | | | | |
|---|---|---|---|---|---|---|---|---|
| 1 | | | | | | 3 | 6 | |
| | | 6 | | | 4 | 1 | 5 | |
| 5 | 3 | 2 | | | 1 | 7 | | |
| | | | | 8 | | | 1 | |
| | | 5 | 9 | | 3 | | 8 | |
| 9 | | | 1 | 2 | 6 | | 7 | |
| 8 | 7 | 9 | | 6 | | | | |
| 3 | | | | 4 | 9 | | | |
| | | | | | | | | |

**Solution on page 117**

# #65

| | | | | | | | | |
|---|---|---|---|---|---|---|---|---|
| | | | | | | | | |
| | | | | 9 | 4 | 2 | | 7 |
| 8 | | | 7 | | | 6 | | |
| | | 7 | | | | | 6 | |
| | | | | | 3 | 9 | | |
| 1 | 8 | | 6 | | 9 | | 3 | |
| | | 5 | | | | | | |
| 2 | | 4 | | | 5 | 3 | 7 | 9 |
| 9 | | | 1 | | | | | |

**Solution on page 118**

# #66

| | | | | | | | | |
|---|---|---|---|---|---|---|---|---|
| | 5 | 1 | | 7 | | 6 | | |
| | | | | | | | | 9 |
| | | 6 | | | | | 2 | |
| | | | | | | 5 | 8 | |
| | | | | 2 | | | 4 | 7 |
| | | 5 | 1 | | 7 | | | |
| 7 | | | | | 5 | | 9 | 8 |
| | 4 | | 2 | 8 | | 7 | | |
| 5 | 6 | 8 | 7 | | | | | 3 |

**Solution on page 118**

# #67

| | 1 | | | | 8 | | | |
|---|---|---|---|---|---|---|---|---|
| | 4 | | 7 | 2 | | 6 | | 1 |
| 6 | | | | | | | | 5 |
| | | 7 | 3 | | | | | |
| 1 | | | 9 | 8 | | | | |
| 3 | | 8 | 1 | | 5 | | 4 | 7 |
| | | | | | | 8 | | |
| | | | | | | | 9 | 3 |
| | 8 | | 2 | | | | 5 | |

**Solution on page 118**

# #68

| | | | | | | | | |
|---|---|---|---|---|---|---|---|---|
| 9 | 5 | | 4 | | | | | 3 |
| 7 | | | | 5 | | 8 | | |
| | | | | | | | 9 | |
| | | | | 7 | | 1 | 2 | 8 |
| | 7 | | 1 | | | | | |
| 5 | 1 | | 9 | | | | 4 | |
| | | 1 | | | 4 | | 6 | 7 |
| | 9 | | | 6 | | | 8 | |
| | 3 | | 8 | | | | | |

**Solution on page 118**

# #69

| | | | | | | | | |
|---|---|---|---|---|---|---|---|---|
| | | | | | | 4 | | |
| 2 | | | | | | | | 6 |
| 9 | | | 5 | | | | | 7 |
| 8 | | | | | | 7 | | 9 |
| | 6 | 9 | 4 | | | 3 | | |
| | 5 | | 6 | 7 | | | 2 | |
| 4 | 2 | | | | | | | |
| | 3 | 7 | 8 | | | 5 | | |
| 5 | | | | | 4 | | 8 | 2 |

**Solution on page 119**

# #70

|  |  |  |  |  |  |  |  |  |
|---|---|---|---|---|---|---|---|---|
|  |  |  |  |  |  |  |  |  |
|  |  |  | 7 | 9 | 2 |  | 6 | 3 |
|  | 1 |  |  | 8 | 6 |  |  |  |
| 1 |  |  |  |  |  | 8 |  |  |
|  | 9 | 8 | 2 | 3 | 5 |  |  |  |
|  | 2 | 5 |  |  |  |  |  | 4 |
|  |  |  |  |  |  | 2 |  | 6 |
|  |  |  | 6 | 2 |  |  | 8 | 9 |
|  |  | 9 |  |  | 3 | 5 | 4 | 1 |

**Solution on page 119**

# #71

| | | | | | | | | |
|---|---|---|---|---|---|---|---|---|
| 4 | | | | 7 | | | 8 | |
| | | | 6 | | | | 5 | 4 |
| | 1 | 3 | | | | | | |
| 2 | 7 | | 1 | | | | | |
| | | | | 2 | | | | |
| | | | | 9 | | 8 | | 6 |
| 7 | 3 | | 4 | | | | | 8 |
| | | | 5 | 8 | 3 | | | |
| | 2 | | | | 9 | 1 | | |

**Solution on page 119**

# #72

| | | | | | | | | |
|---|---|---|---|---|---|---|---|---|
| 8 | | | 9 | 6 | | | | |
| | | | 1 | | | 7 | 5 | 8 |
| | | | | 5 | | | | 6 |
| 1 | 3 | | 8 | | | | | |
| | | | | 4 | 9 | | | |
| | 6 | 7 | | 1 | 5 | | | 9 |
| 2 | | 6 | | | 4 | 9 | | 5 |
| | | 8 | 6 | 2 | | 4 | | 7 |
| | | | | | | | | |

**Solution on page 119**

# #73

| | | | | | | | | |
|---|---|---|---|---|---|---|---|---|
| | | | | | 2 | | 8 | |
| | | 2 | 5 | | 1 | | | |
| 1 | | 6 | 3 | 4 | | | | |
| | 5 | | 4 | 3 | 9 | 7 | | |
| 9 | | | | | 5 | | 4 | 1 |
| | | | 1 | 7 | | | | 6 |
| | | | | | | | | |
| | | 3 | 8 | | | 9 | 1 | |
| | | 9 | | | | 6 | | |

**Solution on page 120**

# #74

| | | | | | | | | |
|---|---|---|---|---|---|---|---|---|
| | 3 | 1 | 8 | | | | 9 | 7 |
| 9 | | | 1 | | 3 | 4 | | 8 |
| 6 | | | | | | | | 1 |
| | | | | | | | | 3 |
| | | | | 9 | 2 | | | |
| | 4 | 3 | 7 | 5 | | | | 6 |
| | | | 9 | | 1 | | 8 | |
| | | | | | | | | 4 |
| | | | 6 | | 7 | 1 | | |

**Solution on page 120**

# #75

| | | | | | | | | |
|---|---|---|---|---|---|---|---|---|
| 2 | | 4 | 3 | | | | | |
| | | 8 | | | | 7 | | 5 |
| | | 6 | | | 1 | | | |
| | | | 4 | | | 2 | | 1 |
| | | | | | 8 | | 7 | |
| 5 | 9 | 7 | | | 2 | | 4 | |
| | | 2 | | | 7 | | 1 | |
| | | | 8 | | 4 | 6 | 5 | |
| | | | | 1 | | 4 | | |

**Solution on page 120**

# #76

| | | | | | | | | |
|---|---|---|---|---|---|---|---|---|
| | | | | | 2 | | 5 | |
| 6 | 8 | | | | 7 | 3 | | |
| 2 | 5 | 1 | 6 | | 3 | | | |
| | | | 3 | | 4 | | | 5 |
| 4 | | 5 | | | | | | |
| | 9 | | | | | | 4 | |
| | | 2 | | 1 | 8 | | 3 | |
| 3 | 1 | | 9 | | | 7 | | |
| | | | 7 | | | 5 | | |

**Solution on page 120**

# #77

| | | | | | | | | |
|---|---|---|---|---|---|---|---|---|
| 6 | | | | | 8 | 5 | | |
| | | 3 | 9 | | 4 | | | |
| 5 | 7 | 9 | 6 | | | | | |
| | | | 4 | | 7 | | | 1 |
| | | | 3 | 8 | | | | 9 |
| | | 7 | | | | | | |
| | | | | | 6 | | 7 | |
| 4 | 3 | | | | 2 | 1 | | 8 |
| | | | 8 | 3 | 5 | | | |

**Solution on page 121**

# #78

| | | | | | | | | |
|---|---|---|---|---|---|---|---|---|
| | 3 | | | | 4 | | 2 | |
| 4 | | | | | 3 | 5 | | |
| 5 | 6 | | 8 | | | | 4 | |
| 8 | 4 | | | | | | | |
| | 1 | 9 | | | | 3 | 5 | |
| | | | | | | | 8 | 9 |
| | | | | 5 | 9 | | | |
| | | 1 | 3 | 7 | | | | 8 |
| | | | | 4 | | | 1 | |

Solution on page 121

# #79

| | | | | | | | | |
|---|---|---|---|---|---|---|---|---|
| 9 | | | 7 | 4 | 1 | | | |
| | | | | | | | 4 | |
| | | | | | | 9 | | 1 |
| | | | 8 | | | | | |
| | 6 | 8 | | | 9 | | 5 | 3 |
| 1 | | | 3 | | | 8 | | |
| | 9 | | | | 4 | 6 | 3 | |
| 3 | 8 | | 9 | | 6 | | | |
| 2 | 1 | | 5 | | 3 | | | |

**Solution on page 121**

# #80

| | | | | | | | | |
|---|---|---|---|---|---|---|---|---|
| | 4 | | | | | | | 9 |
| | | | 1 | 8 | | | | 4 |
| | 2 | 9 | | 3 | | | 5 | |
| | 1 | | | | | | | |
| 9 | | | | 1 | | | 2 | |
| | 7 | | 9 | 4 | 6 | | | |
| | | 8 | | | 3 | 7 | | 6 |
| | | 4 | | | | | | |
| | 3 | 5 | | | | | 9 | |

**Solution on page 121**

# #81

| | | | | | | | | |
|---|---|---|---|---|---|---|---|---|
| | 6 | | | | 1 | | | |
| | | | | 6 | | 7 | 4 | |
| 5 | | | 4 | | | | 1 | |
| 3 | | | | | | | | 2 |
| | | | | 8 | 3 | 9 | 5 | |
| | | | | 7 | 9 | | | |
| | | 8 | | 1 | | 2 | | 6 |
| | | 2 | 7 | | 8 | | | |
| 4 | | 5 | | | | | 9 | |

**Solution on page 122**

# #82

| | | | | | | | | |
|---|---|---|---|---|---|---|---|---|
| 3 | 7 | | | 6 | | | | |
| 1 | | 8 | 5 | | | | | |
| | | 2 | | | | | | 4 |
| | | | | 2 | 8 | | | |
| | | 3 | 4 | 1 | | 8 | 6 | |
| 4 | | | | | | | 7 | |
| | | | 7 | | 2 | | | |
| | 4 | | 6 | | | | | |
| | 2 | 7 | | | 3 | 5 | 8 | |

**Solution on page 122**

# #83

| | | | | | | | | |
|---|---|---|---|---|---|---|---|---|
| | 8 | | | 5 | | | | 2 |
| | | 9 | | | | | 7 | |
| | 5 | 7 | | | | | 3 | |
| | 4 | | 9 | | | | 6 | 7 |
| | | | | | 7 | | | |
| 1 | | 3 | | | | 2 | | |
| 8 | 6 | | 5 | | | 9 | | |
| 3 | | 5 | | | 4 | | | |
| | 1 | | 2 | 3 | | | | 8 |

**Solution on page 122**

# #84

| | | | | | | | | |
|---|---|---|---|---|---|---|---|---|
| 2 | 9 | | 5 | 1 | | | 6 | |
| 1 | 4 | 7 | | | | 3 | | |
| 6 | | | | | | | | |
| 3 | | | | | | | | 4 |
| | | | 3 | | 1 | 6 | 8 | |
| | | | | | | 2 | | |
| 5 | 3 | 6 | 8 | | 4 | | | 2 |
| | 2 | | | | 9 | | | |
| | | 1 | | 3 | 2 | 8 | | |

Solution on page 122

# #85

| | | | | | | | | |
|---|---|---|---|---|---|---|---|---|
| | 1 | | 4 | 8 | | | 7 | |
| | | | | | | | 2 | |
| 8 | | | 3 | | | | | 4 |
| | | | 8 | | 9 | 5 | | |
| 6 | | | | | 3 | | 9 | 2 |
| 5 | | 9 | | | | 7 | 4 | |
| 7 | 2 | 3 | | | | | | 9 |
| | 4 | | | | 6 | | 8 | |
| | | | 2 | | | | | |

Solution on page 123

# #86

|   |   |   |   |   |   |   |   |   |
|---|---|---|---|---|---|---|---|---|
|   | 2 | 8 |   | 6 | 4 |   |   | 3 |
| 6 |   |   |   |   |   | 8 |   |   |
|   |   | 3 |   |   |   |   |   |   |
|   | 7 |   |   | 1 | 6 |   |   | 8 |
|   | 1 |   |   |   |   |   |   | 2 |
|   | 8 |   |   |   | 2 | 1 | 9 | 5 |
| 7 |   | 4 |   | 8 | 9 |   |   | 6 |
| 9 |   |   | 2 | 3 |   |   |   |   |
|   |   |   |   |   |   |   |   | 7 |

**Solution on page 123**

# #87

| | | | | | | | | |
|---|---|---|---|---|---|---|---|---|
| | | | | | 9 | | | |
| | 4 | 1 | | | | 5 | | |
| | | | | 7 | | | | 6 |
| 2 | | 5 | 6 | | 3 | 4 | | |
| 8 | 1 | | 4 | | | | | 2 |
| | 9 | 4 | | 8 | 5 | | | |
| | | 2 | | | | | | |
| | 3 | | | | 8 | | 4 | 7 |
| 7 | | | | | | | 2 | |

**Solution on page 123**

# #88

| | | | | | | | | |
|---|---|---|---|---|---|---|---|---|
| 5 | | | | | 8 | 3 | | |
| | 1 | 2 | | | | 9 | | |
| | | 8 | | 5 | 1 | | | 2 |
| | | 3 | 8 | | | 6 | 9 | |
| 9 | 5 | | 4 | 6 | | | | |
| 7 | | | | | 9 | | | |
| 2 | 7 | | | | | 8 | | |
| | | | | | | 7 | 4 | |
| | 3 | 4 | | | 7 | | | |

**Solution on page 123**

# #89

| | | | | | | | | |
|---|---|---|---|---|---|---|---|---|
| | | 2 | 3 | | | | 1 | 7 |
| | 8 | | | | | | 2 | |
| 3 | | | | | | | | |
| 8 | | | 7 | | 9 | 6 | | |
| | 2 | 3 | 5 | 8 | | | | 9 |
| 6 | | 1 | 2 | | | | | 5 |
| 4 | 5 | | | 9 | | 7 | | |
| | 7 | 6 | | 5 | | 9 | | |
| | | | | | 7 | | | |

**Solution on page 124**

# #90

| | | | | | | | | |
|---|---|---|---|---|---|---|---|---|
| | | | | | | 6 | | |
| 6 | 1 | 7 | | | 5 | | | |
| | | | 9 | | | | 4 | |
| | | 5 | 3 | | | | | |
| 1 | | | | | | 9 | | 8 |
| 3 | | 4 | | | 1 | 7 | 6 | |
| 5 | | | | 9 | | | | |
| 8 | | | | | | | | |
| 4 | | | | 7 | | 8 | 2 | |

**Solution on page 124**

# #91

| | | | | | | | | |
|---|---|---|---|---|---|---|---|---|
| | | 2 | | 4 | | 9 | 3 | |
| | 9 | | | | | 7 | | 4 |
| | | | 2 | | 3 | | | |
| 8 | | 6 | 3 | | | | 9 | |
| 7 | | | | | | | | |
| | | | 6 | | 2 | | | |
| 6 | 7 | | 4 | | 1 | | | |
| | 5 | 4 | | 6 | | 8 | | 2 |
| | | | | | | | | 6 |

**Solution on page 124**

# #92

| | | | | | | | | |
|---|---|---|---|---|---|---|---|---|
| | 5 | | | 2 | | | | 1 |
| 2 | | 8 | | 3 | | | | |
| 6 | | | | | 9 | 2 | | |
| | | | 9 | | | | | |
| 9 | 6 | 3 | | | | | | 8 |
| | | | 6 | 5 | | | | |
| | | | | | 7 | 9 | 5 | |
| | | 5 | | | | 1 | | 4 |
| | 4 | 2 | | | | 7 | 3 | |

**Solution on page 124**

# #93

| | | | | | | | | |
|---|---|---|---|---|---|---|---|---|
| 9 | | | 6 | | 8 | | 2 | |
| | | | 4 | 9 | 5 | | 1 | |
| | | 7 | 3 | | | | | |
| | | | | 2 | | | | |
| 6 | | 3 | | 5 | | | 9 | |
| | 4 | | | | | | | 5 |
| 5 | 3 | 2 | | | 1 | | | 4 |
| | | 9 | | | | | 3 | 1 |
| 4 | | | | | | | | |

**Solution on page 125**

# #94

| | | | | | | | | |
|---|---|---|---|---|---|---|---|---|
| | | | | | | | | |
| | 3 | 4 | | 8 | 1 | | | 5 |
| 6 | 1 | | | | 3 | 9 | | |
| | | | 3 | 2 | 6 | | | |
| | 7 | 9 | 8 | | | | | |
| | 5 | 6 | | | | | 4 | |
| 8 | | | 1 | | | 6 | | |
| | 6 | 1 | | 9 | | 3 | | |
| | | 3 | | | 5 | | | 1 |

**Solution on page 125**

# #95

| | | | | | | | | |
|---|---|---|---|---|---|---|---|---|
| 3 | | 9 | 4 | | | | | |
| | | | | 9 | 7 | 5 | | |
| | | 2 | 6 | | | 4 | 9 | |
| | 6 | | | | | | 4 | 2 |
| | | 8 | 2 | | | | 5 | |
| | | | | | | 7 | 6 | |
| 8 | | 1 | | | | | 7 | |
| | 2 | | | | 4 | | 8 | |
| 9 | | | | | 5 | 2 | | |

Solution on page 125

# #96

| | | | | | | | | |
|---|---|---|---|---|---|---|---|---|
| 7 | 5 | | | | 1 | | | 8 |
| | 4 | | | | | 5 | | 1 |
| 3 | 1 | | 8 | | | | | |
| | 7 | | 2 | | | | 3 | 4 |
| 1 | | | | 8 | | 2 | | |
| | | 3 | 9 | | | 8 | | |
| 4 | | | | 7 | | | 5 | |
| | | 2 | | | | 4 | | |
| 5 | | | | | | | | |

**Solution on page 125**

# #97

| | | | | | | | | |
|---|---|---|---|---|---|---|---|---|
| 6 | 3 | | 1 | | | | | |
| | | | 5 | | | | | |
| | | | | | 8 | 2 | | |
| | | | 2 | 9 | | | | |
| | 5 | 3 | | | | 4 | | 9 |
| 1 | | 6 | | | | | 2 | |
| | | 2 | | 5 | | | | 1 |
| | | 5 | | | 6 | 9 | | 3 |
| | 6 | | 8 | 3 | | 5 | | 2 |

**Solution on page 126**

# #98

| | | | | | | | | |
|---|---|---|---|---|---|---|---|---|
| 2 | 8 | | | 4 | | 1 | | |
| | | 5 | | | | | | |
| | | 6 | | 1 | 5 | 2 | 8 | |
| 5 | | | 1 | 2 | | | 9 | |
| 9 | 4 | | 5 | 7 | 6 | | | |
| | 2 | | | | | | 6 | |
| | | | | 8 | | 3 | | 9 |
| | 9 | | | | | | | |
| 8 | | 3 | 4 | | | | 1 | |

**Solution on page 126**

# #99

| | | | | | | | | |
|---|---|---|---|---|---|---|---|---|
| 1 | | | | | | | 8 | |
| 2 | | | 4 | | | | 3 | |
| | 7 | | | | | | 4 | 6 |
| | | 3 | | | 6 | 7 | 9 | 4 |
| 4 | | | 7 | | | | | |
| 8 | | | | | | | | 5 |
| | 1 | | | | | | | |
| | | | | 6 | | | | 9 |
| | | 4 | | | 5 | | 2 | 3 |

**Solution on page 126**

# #100

| | | | | | | | | |
|---|---|---|---|---|---|---|---|---|
| | 7 | 2 | | | | 4 | | |
| 9 | 6 | | | | 2 | 1 | | |
| | | 3 | 4 | | | | | |
| 4 | | 9 | | | 1 | | 2 | 6 |
| | | | | 2 | 8 | | | |
| | 8 | 6 | | | | | | |
| 6 | | | | 9 | | | 8 | 4 |
| | | | | 3 | 6 | | | 7 |
| | | | 2 | | | | 1 | |

**Solution on page 126**

## #1

| | | | | | | | | |
|---|---|---|---|---|---|---|---|---|
| 7 | 1 | 6 | 3 | 9 | 5 | 8 | 2 | 4 |
| 4 | 8 | 3 | 2 | 1 | 6 | 9 | 7 | 5 |
| 2 | 5 | 9 | 7 | 8 | 4 | 6 | 3 | 1 |
| 8 | 4 | 5 | 6 | 7 | 1 | 2 | 9 | 3 |
| 1 | 6 | 2 | 9 | 3 | 8 | 5 | 4 | 7 |
| 3 | 9 | 7 | 4 | 5 | 2 | 1 | 6 | 8 |
| 5 | 7 | 4 | 8 | 2 | 9 | 3 | 1 | 6 |
| 6 | 2 | 8 | 1 | 4 | 3 | 7 | 5 | 9 |
| 9 | 3 | 1 | 5 | 6 | 7 | 4 | 8 | 2 |

## #2

| | | | | | | | | |
|---|---|---|---|---|---|---|---|---|
| 8 | 6 | 1 | 3 | 4 | 9 | 5 | 2 | 7 |
| 7 | 5 | 3 | 6 | 8 | 2 | 4 | 1 | 9 |
| 9 | 2 | 4 | 5 | 1 | 7 | 6 | 8 | 3 |
| 3 | 8 | 7 | 1 | 5 | 4 | 9 | 6 | 2 |
| 5 | 4 | 2 | 9 | 7 | 6 | 8 | 3 | 1 |
| 1 | 9 | 6 | 8 | 2 | 3 | 7 | 4 | 5 |
| 4 | 3 | 8 | 2 | 9 | 5 | 1 | 7 | 6 |
| 6 | 7 | 5 | 4 | 3 | 1 | 2 | 9 | 8 |
| 2 | 1 | 9 | 7 | 6 | 8 | 3 | 5 | 4 |

## #3

| | | | | | | | | |
|---|---|---|---|---|---|---|---|---|
| 8 | 5 | 6 | 3 | 7 | 2 | 1 | 9 | 4 |
| 2 | 1 | 7 | 4 | 6 | 9 | 5 | 8 | 3 |
| 4 | 9 | 3 | 5 | 8 | 1 | 7 | 2 | 6 |
| 6 | 3 | 2 | 8 | 1 | 7 | 4 | 5 | 9 |
| 9 | 4 | 8 | 6 | 5 | 3 | 2 | 7 | 1 |
| 1 | 7 | 5 | 2 | 9 | 4 | 6 | 3 | 8 |
| 3 | 6 | 9 | 7 | 4 | 5 | 8 | 1 | 2 |
| 5 | 2 | 4 | 1 | 3 | 8 | 9 | 6 | 7 |
| 7 | 8 | 1 | 9 | 2 | 6 | 3 | 4 | 5 |

## #4

| | | | | | | | | |
|---|---|---|---|---|---|---|---|---|
| 9 | 4 | 2 | 3 | 1 | 6 | 5 | 8 | 7 |
| 3 | 6 | 5 | 8 | 7 | 9 | 4 | 1 | 2 |
| 1 | 8 | 7 | 2 | 5 | 4 | 6 | 9 | 3 |
| 8 | 5 | 1 | 7 | 4 | 2 | 9 | 3 | 6 |
| 6 | 2 | 4 | 9 | 3 | 8 | 7 | 5 | 1 |
| 7 | 9 | 3 | 1 | 6 | 5 | 2 | 4 | 8 |
| 2 | 3 | 8 | 4 | 9 | 7 | 1 | 6 | 5 |
| 5 | 7 | 9 | 6 | 8 | 1 | 3 | 2 | 4 |
| 4 | 1 | 6 | 5 | 2 | 3 | 8 | 7 | 9 |

## #5

| | | | | | | | | |
|---|---|---|---|---|---|---|---|---|
| 3 | 1 | 6 | 4 | 7 | 5 | 2 | 9 | 8 |
| 5 | 9 | 2 | 1 | 6 | 8 | 4 | 3 | 7 |
| 7 | 4 | 8 | 9 | 3 | 2 | 5 | 6 | 1 |
| 2 | 6 | 7 | 3 | 5 | 9 | 1 | 8 | 4 |
| 1 | 5 | 3 | 2 | 8 | 4 | 9 | 7 | 6 |
| 4 | 8 | 9 | 6 | 1 | 7 | 3 | 5 | 2 |
| 6 | 3 | 5 | 7 | 2 | 1 | 8 | 4 | 9 |
| 9 | 7 | 1 | 8 | 4 | 3 | 6 | 2 | 5 |
| 8 | 2 | 4 | 5 | 9 | 6 | 7 | 1 | 3 |

## #6

| | | | | | | | | |
|---|---|---|---|---|---|---|---|---|
| 7 | 4 | 6 | 3 | 2 | 1 | 5 | 9 | 8 |
| 2 | 8 | 3 | 9 | 5 | 6 | 7 | 1 | 4 |
| 1 | 5 | 9 | 8 | 4 | 7 | 6 | 3 | 2 |
| 8 | 1 | 5 | 7 | 6 | 4 | 3 | 2 | 9 |
| 6 | 9 | 4 | 2 | 3 | 5 | 8 | 7 | 1 |
| 3 | 2 | 7 | 1 | 9 | 8 | 4 | 6 | 5 |
| 4 | 7 | 1 | 6 | 8 | 9 | 2 | 5 | 3 |
| 5 | 6 | 2 | 4 | 1 | 3 | 9 | 8 | 7 |
| 9 | 3 | 8 | 5 | 7 | 2 | 1 | 4 | 6 |

## #7

| | | | | | | | | |
|---|---|---|---|---|---|---|---|---|
| 8 | 6 | 4 | 5 | 9 | 1 | 7 | 3 | 2 |
| 5 | 9 | 2 | 6 | 7 | 3 | 1 | 8 | 4 |
| 7 | 3 | 1 | 2 | 8 | 4 | 9 | 6 | 5 |
| 9 | 2 | 8 | 1 | 3 | 7 | 5 | 4 | 6 |
| 3 | 4 | 5 | 9 | 6 | 8 | 2 | 1 | 7 |
| 6 | 1 | 7 | 4 | 5 | 2 | 3 | 9 | 8 |
| 2 | 7 | 6 | 8 | 1 | 9 | 4 | 5 | 3 |
| 4 | 5 | 9 | 3 | 2 | 6 | 8 | 7 | 1 |
| 1 | 8 | 3 | 7 | 4 | 5 | 6 | 2 | 9 |

## #8

| | | | | | | | | |
|---|---|---|---|---|---|---|---|---|
| 5 | 3 | 4 | 2 | 6 | 8 | 1 | 7 | 9 |
| 8 | 2 | 7 | 9 | 1 | 3 | 5 | 4 | 6 |
| 1 | 6 | 9 | 7 | 5 | 4 | 8 | 3 | 2 |
| 7 | 8 | 2 | 6 | 9 | 5 | 3 | 1 | 4 |
| 4 | 5 | 1 | 3 | 8 | 2 | 6 | 9 | 7 |
| 6 | 9 | 3 | 1 | 4 | 7 | 2 | 8 | 5 |
| 9 | 7 | 6 | 5 | 3 | 1 | 4 | 2 | 8 |
| 3 | 4 | 5 | 8 | 2 | 9 | 7 | 6 | 1 |
| 2 | 1 | 8 | 4 | 7 | 6 | 9 | 5 | 3 |

# #9

| 3 | 4 | 8 | 9 | 1 | 2 | 5 | 6 | 7 |
|---|---|---|---|---|---|---|---|---|
| 7 | 2 | 5 | 4 | 3 | 6 | 9 | 1 | 8 |
| 9 | 1 | 6 | 7 | 5 | 8 | 3 | 2 | 4 |
| 6 | 9 | 2 | 8 | 7 | 3 | 1 | 4 | 5 |
| 1 | 7 | 3 | 5 | 9 | 4 | 6 | 8 | 2 |
| 5 | 8 | 4 | 2 | 6 | 1 | 7 | 3 | 9 |
| 2 | 6 | 9 | 1 | 8 | 5 | 4 | 7 | 3 |
| 8 | 3 | 7 | 6 | 4 | 9 | 2 | 5 | 1 |
| 4 | 5 | 1 | 3 | 2 | 7 | 8 | 9 | 6 |

# #10

| 2 | 7 | 9 | 6 | 8 | 5 | 4 | 1 | 3 |
|---|---|---|---|---|---|---|---|---|
| 1 | 3 | 8 | 2 | 9 | 4 | 5 | 6 | 7 |
| 6 | 5 | 4 | 3 | 7 | 1 | 8 | 2 | 9 |
| 7 | 9 | 3 | 5 | 4 | 2 | 6 | 8 | 1 |
| 4 | 1 | 2 | 9 | 6 | 8 | 3 | 7 | 5 |
| 5 | 8 | 6 | 1 | 3 | 7 | 9 | 4 | 2 |
| 8 | 2 | 1 | 4 | 5 | 9 | 7 | 3 | 6 |
| 9 | 6 | 7 | 8 | 2 | 3 | 1 | 5 | 4 |
| 3 | 4 | 5 | 7 | 1 | 6 | 2 | 9 | 8 |

# #11

| 4 | 6 | 8 | 9 | 5 | 1 | 7 | 2 | 3 |
|---|---|---|---|---|---|---|---|---|
| 7 | 3 | 5 | 2 | 4 | 8 | 6 | 9 | 1 |
| 2 | 1 | 9 | 3 | 6 | 7 | 5 | 4 | 8 |
| 5 | 7 | 3 | 8 | 9 | 2 | 4 | 1 | 6 |
| 9 | 2 | 6 | 4 | 1 | 3 | 8 | 5 | 7 |
| 8 | 4 | 1 | 5 | 7 | 6 | 2 | 3 | 9 |
| 3 | 8 | 7 | 1 | 2 | 5 | 9 | 6 | 4 |
| 6 | 9 | 2 | 7 | 3 | 4 | 1 | 8 | 5 |
| 1 | 5 | 4 | 6 | 8 | 9 | 3 | 7 | 2 |

# #12

| 8 | 4 | 9 | 6 | 5 | 2 | 1 | 3 | 7 |
|---|---|---|---|---|---|---|---|---|
| 1 | 2 | 6 | 8 | 3 | 7 | 4 | 5 | 9 |
| 5 | 7 | 3 | 9 | 4 | 1 | 2 | 8 | 6 |
| 9 | 5 | 2 | 4 | 7 | 6 | 8 | 1 | 3 |
| 6 | 1 | 7 | 5 | 8 | 3 | 9 | 4 | 2 |
| 4 | 3 | 8 | 1 | 2 | 9 | 7 | 6 | 5 |
| 3 | 9 | 5 | 2 | 1 | 4 | 6 | 7 | 8 |
| 2 | 8 | 4 | 7 | 6 | 5 | 3 | 9 | 1 |
| 7 | 6 | 1 | 3 | 9 | 8 | 5 | 2 | 4 |

# #13

| | | | | | | | | |
|---|---|---|---|---|---|---|---|---|
| 4 | 6 | 5 | 3 | 1 | 2 | 8 | 7 | 9 |
| 1 | 7 | 8 | 5 | 4 | 9 | 6 | 2 | 3 |
| 9 | 2 | 3 | 7 | 8 | 6 | 4 | 1 | 5 |
| 7 | 4 | 2 | 1 | 5 | 8 | 9 | 3 | 6 |
| 5 | 1 | 9 | 6 | 7 | 3 | 2 | 8 | 4 |
| 3 | 8 | 6 | 2 | 9 | 4 | 1 | 5 | 7 |
| 8 | 3 | 7 | 4 | 6 | 1 | 5 | 9 | 2 |
| 6 | 5 | 1 | 9 | 2 | 7 | 3 | 4 | 8 |
| 2 | 9 | 4 | 8 | 3 | 5 | 7 | 6 | 1 |

# #14

| | | | | | | | | |
|---|---|---|---|---|---|---|---|---|
| 8 | 4 | 1 | 6 | 2 | 7 | 9 | 3 | 5 |
| 9 | 5 | 7 | 1 | 8 | 3 | 6 | 4 | 2 |
| 6 | 3 | 2 | 9 | 5 | 4 | 7 | 8 | 1 |
| 4 | 1 | 9 | 3 | 6 | 2 | 8 | 5 | 7 |
| 3 | 8 | 6 | 5 | 7 | 9 | 2 | 1 | 4 |
| 7 | 2 | 5 | 8 | 4 | 1 | 3 | 9 | 6 |
| 2 | 6 | 8 | 4 | 9 | 5 | 1 | 7 | 3 |
| 5 | 9 | 3 | 7 | 1 | 6 | 4 | 2 | 8 |
| 1 | 7 | 4 | 2 | 3 | 8 | 5 | 6 | 9 |

# #15

| | | | | | | | | |
|---|---|---|---|---|---|---|---|---|
| 8 | 9 | 3 | 5 | 1 | 4 | 6 | 7 | 2 |
| 5 | 1 | 2 | 8 | 6 | 7 | 4 | 3 | 9 |
| 7 | 6 | 4 | 2 | 3 | 9 | 5 | 8 | 1 |
| 1 | 4 | 7 | 9 | 5 | 8 | 3 | 2 | 6 |
| 9 | 5 | 6 | 3 | 7 | 2 | 8 | 1 | 4 |
| 2 | 3 | 8 | 6 | 4 | 1 | 7 | 9 | 5 |
| 3 | 7 | 5 | 1 | 9 | 6 | 2 | 4 | 8 |
| 6 | 2 | 1 | 4 | 8 | 3 | 9 | 5 | 7 |
| 4 | 8 | 9 | 7 | 2 | 5 | 1 | 6 | 3 |

# #16

| | | | | | | | | |
|---|---|---|---|---|---|---|---|---|
| 4 | 8 | 5 | 9 | 2 | 3 | 1 | 7 | 6 |
| 9 | 3 | 7 | 1 | 4 | 6 | 5 | 2 | 8 |
| 6 | 2 | 1 | 5 | 8 | 7 | 3 | 9 | 4 |
| 8 | 4 | 9 | 7 | 3 | 1 | 2 | 6 | 5 |
| 7 | 5 | 6 | 8 | 9 | 2 | 4 | 3 | 1 |
| 2 | 1 | 3 | 6 | 5 | 4 | 9 | 8 | 7 |
| 5 | 6 | 8 | 3 | 1 | 9 | 7 | 4 | 2 |
| 1 | 9 | 4 | 2 | 7 | 8 | 6 | 5 | 3 |
| 3 | 7 | 2 | 4 | 6 | 5 | 8 | 1 | 9 |

# #17

| 1 | 4 | 5 | 2 | 9 | 6 | 7 | 8 | 3 |
|---|---|---|---|---|---|---|---|---|
| 2 | 6 | 7 | 8 | 3 | 1 | 4 | 5 | 9 |
| 9 | 8 | 3 | 7 | 5 | 4 | 6 | 2 | 1 |
| 7 | 2 | 1 | 4 | 8 | 9 | 5 | 3 | 6 |
| 6 | 3 | 9 | 5 | 1 | 2 | 8 | 7 | 4 |
| 8 | 5 | 4 | 6 | 7 | 3 | 1 | 9 | 2 |
| 3 | 1 | 8 | 9 | 6 | 5 | 2 | 4 | 7 |
| 4 | 7 | 6 | 3 | 2 | 8 | 9 | 1 | 5 |
| 5 | 9 | 2 | 1 | 4 | 7 | 3 | 6 | 8 |

# #18

| 4 | 8 | 2 | 7 | 1 | 9 | 3 | 5 | 6 |
|---|---|---|---|---|---|---|---|---|
| 1 | 3 | 5 | 2 | 6 | 8 | 7 | 9 | 4 |
| 9 | 7 | 6 | 4 | 3 | 5 | 8 | 2 | 1 |
| 6 | 5 | 9 | 3 | 4 | 7 | 1 | 8 | 2 |
| 3 | 4 | 7 | 8 | 2 | 1 | 5 | 6 | 9 |
| 8 | 2 | 1 | 5 | 9 | 6 | 4 | 3 | 7 |
| 7 | 1 | 3 | 6 | 5 | 2 | 9 | 4 | 8 |
| 5 | 6 | 8 | 9 | 7 | 4 | 2 | 1 | 3 |
| 2 | 9 | 4 | 1 | 8 | 3 | 6 | 7 | 5 |

# #19

| 9 | 7 | 8 | 1 | 4 | 3 | 5 | 2 | 6 |
|---|---|---|---|---|---|---|---|---|
| 6 | 5 | 3 | 9 | 2 | 8 | 4 | 7 | 1 |
| 4 | 1 | 2 | 7 | 6 | 5 | 3 | 8 | 9 |
| 5 | 9 | 4 | 6 | 8 | 7 | 1 | 3 | 2 |
| 3 | 6 | 7 | 2 | 9 | 1 | 8 | 4 | 5 |
| 8 | 2 | 1 | 5 | 3 | 4 | 6 | 9 | 7 |
| 1 | 3 | 9 | 8 | 5 | 2 | 7 | 6 | 4 |
| 7 | 8 | 6 | 4 | 1 | 9 | 2 | 5 | 3 |
| 2 | 4 | 5 | 3 | 7 | 6 | 9 | 1 | 8 |

# #20

| 1 | 5 | 3 | 4 | 7 | 6 | 8 | 9 | 2 |
|---|---|---|---|---|---|---|---|---|
| 7 | 9 | 6 | 5 | 2 | 8 | 1 | 3 | 4 |
| 2 | 4 | 8 | 9 | 1 | 3 | 7 | 5 | 6 |
| 8 | 7 | 9 | 2 | 5 | 4 | 6 | 1 | 3 |
| 4 | 6 | 5 | 7 | 3 | 1 | 2 | 8 | 9 |
| 3 | 1 | 2 | 6 | 8 | 9 | 5 | 4 | 7 |
| 5 | 8 | 4 | 3 | 6 | 2 | 9 | 7 | 1 |
| 6 | 3 | 7 | 1 | 9 | 5 | 4 | 2 | 8 |
| 9 | 2 | 1 | 8 | 4 | 7 | 3 | 6 | 5 |

# #21

| | | | | | | | | |
|---|---|---|---|---|---|---|---|---|
| 4 | 3 | 2 | 8 | 1 | 5 | 6 | 7 | 9 |
| 6 | 9 | 1 | 4 | 7 | 3 | 5 | 2 | 8 |
| 8 | 7 | 5 | 6 | 9 | 2 | 1 | 4 | 3 |
| 2 | 4 | 7 | 3 | 6 | 8 | 9 | 1 | 5 |
| 9 | 6 | 3 | 1 | 5 | 4 | 2 | 8 | 7 |
| 1 | 5 | 8 | 7 | 2 | 9 | 3 | 6 | 4 |
| 3 | 1 | 6 | 9 | 8 | 7 | 4 | 5 | 2 |
| 5 | 8 | 9 | 2 | 4 | 6 | 7 | 3 | 1 |
| 7 | 2 | 4 | 5 | 3 | 1 | 8 | 9 | 6 |

# #22

| | | | | | | | | |
|---|---|---|---|---|---|---|---|---|
| 8 | 6 | 4 | 9 | 5 | 3 | 7 | 1 | 2 |
| 9 | 3 | 7 | 2 | 6 | 1 | 4 | 8 | 5 |
| 5 | 2 | 1 | 4 | 8 | 7 | 3 | 6 | 9 |
| 7 | 5 | 8 | 6 | 2 | 9 | 1 | 3 | 4 |
| 3 | 4 | 2 | 7 | 1 | 5 | 8 | 9 | 6 |
| 1 | 9 | 6 | 3 | 4 | 8 | 5 | 2 | 7 |
| 6 | 1 | 3 | 5 | 7 | 2 | 9 | 4 | 8 |
| 4 | 7 | 9 | 8 | 3 | 6 | 2 | 5 | 1 |
| 2 | 8 | 5 | 1 | 9 | 4 | 6 | 7 | 3 |

# #23

| | | | | | | | | |
|---|---|---|---|---|---|---|---|---|
| 7 | 1 | 2 | 3 | 8 | 5 | 6 | 4 | 9 |
| 3 | 9 | 6 | 4 | 7 | 1 | 5 | 2 | 8 |
| 5 | 4 | 8 | 9 | 2 | 6 | 1 | 7 | 3 |
| 1 | 8 | 5 | 7 | 3 | 4 | 2 | 9 | 6 |
| 4 | 2 | 3 | 8 | 6 | 9 | 7 | 1 | 5 |
| 9 | 6 | 7 | 5 | 1 | 2 | 3 | 8 | 4 |
| 2 | 3 | 1 | 6 | 4 | 8 | 9 | 5 | 7 |
| 6 | 5 | 4 | 1 | 9 | 7 | 8 | 3 | 2 |
| 8 | 7 | 9 | 2 | 5 | 3 | 4 | 6 | 1 |

# #24

| | | | | | | | | |
|---|---|---|---|---|---|---|---|---|
| 5 | 1 | 6 | 7 | 8 | 4 | 3 | 2 | 9 |
| 4 | 7 | 9 | 3 | 6 | 2 | 1 | 8 | 5 |
| 2 | 8 | 3 | 1 | 9 | 5 | 7 | 6 | 4 |
| 6 | 4 | 8 | 5 | 7 | 3 | 9 | 1 | 2 |
| 9 | 2 | 7 | 8 | 1 | 6 | 5 | 4 | 3 |
| 3 | 5 | 1 | 2 | 4 | 9 | 8 | 7 | 6 |
| 8 | 6 | 5 | 9 | 2 | 7 | 4 | 3 | 1 |
| 7 | 9 | 4 | 6 | 3 | 1 | 2 | 5 | 8 |
| 1 | 3 | 2 | 4 | 5 | 8 | 6 | 9 | 7 |

## #25

| | | | | | | | | |
|---|---|---|---|---|---|---|---|---|
| 5 | 2 | 6 | 3 | 1 | 9 | 8 | 4 | 7 |
| 3 | 8 | 4 | 5 | 7 | 6 | 2 | 9 | 1 |
| 9 | 7 | 1 | 2 | 8 | 4 | 6 | 5 | 3 |
| 1 | 9 | 3 | 8 | 4 | 2 | 7 | 6 | 5 |
| 8 | 4 | 5 | 6 | 3 | 7 | 9 | 1 | 2 |
| 2 | 6 | 7 | 1 | 9 | 5 | 3 | 8 | 4 |
| 6 | 1 | 9 | 7 | 5 | 3 | 4 | 2 | 8 |
| 4 | 3 | 8 | 9 | 2 | 1 | 5 | 7 | 6 |
| 7 | 5 | 2 | 4 | 6 | 8 | 1 | 3 | 9 |

## #26

| | | | | | | | | |
|---|---|---|---|---|---|---|---|---|
| 9 | 2 | 4 | 5 | 3 | 8 | 7 | 6 | 1 |
| 1 | 7 | 5 | 6 | 9 | 2 | 4 | 8 | 3 |
| 6 | 3 | 8 | 1 | 7 | 4 | 5 | 2 | 9 |
| 8 | 1 | 3 | 7 | 6 | 9 | 2 | 4 | 5 |
| 4 | 9 | 7 | 2 | 5 | 1 | 8 | 3 | 6 |
| 5 | 6 | 2 | 8 | 4 | 3 | 9 | 1 | 7 |
| 3 | 4 | 6 | 9 | 2 | 5 | 1 | 7 | 8 |
| 7 | 8 | 9 | 4 | 1 | 6 | 3 | 5 | 2 |
| 2 | 5 | 1 | 3 | 8 | 7 | 6 | 9 | 4 |

## #27

| | | | | | | | | |
|---|---|---|---|---|---|---|---|---|
| 1 | 9 | 6 | 5 | 2 | 7 | 3 | 8 | 4 |
| 5 | 7 | 2 | 3 | 8 | 4 | 9 | 1 | 6 |
| 8 | 3 | 4 | 6 | 1 | 9 | 5 | 7 | 2 |
| 2 | 6 | 1 | 8 | 3 | 5 | 7 | 4 | 9 |
| 4 | 8 | 7 | 9 | 6 | 1 | 2 | 3 | 5 |
| 3 | 5 | 9 | 7 | 4 | 2 | 1 | 6 | 8 |
| 7 | 2 | 3 | 4 | 9 | 8 | 6 | 5 | 1 |
| 6 | 1 | 8 | 2 | 5 | 3 | 4 | 9 | 7 |
| 9 | 4 | 5 | 1 | 7 | 6 | 8 | 2 | 3 |

## #28

| | | | | | | | | |
|---|---|---|---|---|---|---|---|---|
| 6 | 5 | 1 | 9 | 7 | 2 | 4 | 8 | 3 |
| 3 | 9 | 2 | 8 | 4 | 5 | 6 | 1 | 7 |
| 7 | 4 | 8 | 6 | 1 | 3 | 2 | 5 | 9 |
| 9 | 6 | 3 | 2 | 5 | 1 | 7 | 4 | 8 |
| 1 | 8 | 5 | 4 | 6 | 7 | 3 | 9 | 2 |
| 4 | 2 | 7 | 3 | 8 | 9 | 5 | 6 | 1 |
| 8 | 7 | 9 | 5 | 3 | 6 | 1 | 2 | 4 |
| 5 | 1 | 4 | 7 | 2 | 8 | 9 | 3 | 6 |
| 2 | 3 | 6 | 1 | 9 | 4 | 8 | 7 | 5 |

## #29

| | | | | | | | | |
|---|---|---|---|---|---|---|---|---|
| 3 | 9 | 5 | 4 | 8 | 6 | 1 | 2 | 7 |
| 6 | 4 | 2 | 3 | 1 | 7 | 9 | 8 | 5 |
| 8 | 7 | 1 | 9 | 5 | 2 | 4 | 6 | 3 |
| 5 | 3 | 7 | 2 | 9 | 1 | 6 | 4 | 8 |
| 2 | 6 | 9 | 8 | 4 | 3 | 5 | 7 | 1 |
| 1 | 8 | 4 | 7 | 6 | 5 | 3 | 9 | 2 |
| 4 | 5 | 3 | 6 | 2 | 8 | 7 | 1 | 9 |
| 7 | 2 | 6 | 1 | 3 | 9 | 8 | 5 | 4 |
| 9 | 1 | 8 | 5 | 7 | 4 | 2 | 3 | 6 |

## #30

| | | | | | | | | |
|---|---|---|---|---|---|---|---|---|
| 8 | 5 | 7 | 1 | 2 | 9 | 4 | 6 | 3 |
| 1 | 3 | 6 | 4 | 8 | 5 | 9 | 7 | 2 |
| 4 | 2 | 9 | 3 | 6 | 7 | 8 | 5 | 1 |
| 3 | 9 | 8 | 6 | 1 | 2 | 7 | 4 | 5 |
| 6 | 7 | 4 | 8 | 5 | 3 | 1 | 2 | 9 |
| 2 | 1 | 5 | 9 | 7 | 4 | 6 | 3 | 8 |
| 7 | 8 | 1 | 2 | 3 | 6 | 5 | 9 | 4 |
| 5 | 4 | 3 | 7 | 9 | 8 | 2 | 1 | 6 |
| 9 | 6 | 2 | 5 | 4 | 1 | 3 | 8 | 7 |

## #31

| | | | | | | | | |
|---|---|---|---|---|---|---|---|---|
| 6 | 8 | 7 | 5 | 1 | 3 | 4 | 2 | 9 |
| 3 | 1 | 9 | 7 | 4 | 2 | 6 | 5 | 8 |
| 5 | 2 | 4 | 8 | 9 | 6 | 7 | 1 | 3 |
| 8 | 7 | 6 | 2 | 3 | 4 | 1 | 9 | 5 |
| 2 | 4 | 1 | 6 | 5 | 9 | 8 | 3 | 7 |
| 9 | 3 | 5 | 1 | 7 | 8 | 2 | 6 | 4 |
| 1 | 5 | 2 | 9 | 8 | 7 | 3 | 4 | 6 |
| 7 | 9 | 3 | 4 | 6 | 1 | 5 | 8 | 2 |
| 4 | 6 | 8 | 3 | 2 | 5 | 9 | 7 | 1 |

## #32

| | | | | | | | | |
|---|---|---|---|---|---|---|---|---|
| 3 | 6 | 7 | 5 | 1 | 9 | 2 | 8 | 4 |
| 8 | 5 | 2 | 3 | 4 | 6 | 7 | 1 | 9 |
| 1 | 9 | 4 | 7 | 2 | 8 | 5 | 3 | 6 |
| 5 | 4 | 9 | 1 | 7 | 2 | 8 | 6 | 3 |
| 2 | 8 | 6 | 9 | 3 | 4 | 1 | 5 | 7 |
| 7 | 3 | 1 | 6 | 8 | 5 | 4 | 9 | 2 |
| 4 | 1 | 5 | 2 | 9 | 3 | 6 | 7 | 8 |
| 6 | 2 | 3 | 8 | 5 | 7 | 9 | 4 | 1 |
| 9 | 7 | 8 | 4 | 6 | 1 | 3 | 2 | 5 |

# #33

| 3 | 5 | 6 | 8 | 1 | 2 | 4 | 7 | 9 |
|---|---|---|---|---|---|---|---|---|
| 4 | 7 | 2 | 6 | 5 | 9 | 1 | 3 | 8 |
| 1 | 9 | 8 | 7 | 4 | 3 | 5 | 6 | 2 |
| 8 | 3 | 7 | 5 | 9 | 6 | 2 | 1 | 4 |
| 2 | 1 | 5 | 3 | 8 | 4 | 6 | 9 | 7 |
| 9 | 6 | 4 | 2 | 7 | 1 | 3 | 8 | 5 |
| 5 | 2 | 9 | 1 | 3 | 8 | 7 | 4 | 6 |
| 7 | 8 | 3 | 4 | 6 | 5 | 9 | 2 | 1 |
| 6 | 4 | 1 | 9 | 2 | 7 | 8 | 5 | 3 |

# #34

| 4 | 6 | 5 | 1 | 2 | 3 | 9 | 8 | 7 |
|---|---|---|---|---|---|---|---|---|
| 7 | 8 | 1 | 4 | 6 | 9 | 3 | 2 | 5 |
| 9 | 2 | 3 | 8 | 7 | 5 | 4 | 1 | 6 |
| 6 | 1 | 2 | 9 | 5 | 4 | 7 | 3 | 8 |
| 8 | 3 | 4 | 7 | 1 | 6 | 5 | 9 | 2 |
| 5 | 7 | 9 | 3 | 8 | 2 | 6 | 4 | 1 |
| 1 | 4 | 6 | 5 | 3 | 8 | 2 | 7 | 9 |
| 2 | 9 | 7 | 6 | 4 | 1 | 8 | 5 | 3 |
| 3 | 5 | 8 | 2 | 9 | 7 | 1 | 6 | 4 |

# #35

| 9 | 1 | 4 | 2 | 8 | 5 | 7 | 6 | 3 |
|---|---|---|---|---|---|---|---|---|
| 2 | 7 | 3 | 6 | 1 | 9 | 8 | 5 | 4 |
| 5 | 8 | 6 | 4 | 7 | 3 | 2 | 1 | 9 |
| 6 | 3 | 8 | 5 | 2 | 7 | 9 | 4 | 1 |
| 4 | 2 | 1 | 8 | 9 | 6 | 5 | 3 | 7 |
| 7 | 5 | 9 | 1 | 3 | 4 | 6 | 8 | 2 |
| 1 | 4 | 2 | 7 | 5 | 8 | 3 | 9 | 6 |
| 3 | 6 | 5 | 9 | 4 | 2 | 1 | 7 | 8 |
| 8 | 9 | 7 | 3 | 6 | 1 | 4 | 2 | 5 |

# #36

| 4 | 5 | 7 | 9 | 3 | 6 | 1 | 8 | 2 |
|---|---|---|---|---|---|---|---|---|
| 6 | 2 | 8 | 1 | 5 | 7 | 4 | 9 | 3 |
| 1 | 3 | 9 | 4 | 8 | 2 | 7 | 6 | 5 |
| 5 | 1 | 6 | 8 | 9 | 4 | 3 | 2 | 7 |
| 7 | 4 | 3 | 2 | 6 | 1 | 8 | 5 | 9 |
| 9 | 8 | 2 | 5 | 7 | 3 | 6 | 4 | 1 |
| 3 | 9 | 4 | 6 | 1 | 5 | 2 | 7 | 8 |
| 2 | 7 | 5 | 3 | 4 | 8 | 9 | 1 | 6 |
| 8 | 6 | 1 | 7 | 2 | 9 | 5 | 3 | 4 |

# #37

| | | | | | | | | |
|---|---|---|---|---|---|---|---|---|
| 5 | 7 | 1 | 2 | 3 | 9 | 4 | 6 | 8 |
| 4 | 9 | 6 | 1 | 7 | 8 | 2 | 5 | 3 |
| 3 | 8 | 2 | 5 | 4 | 6 | 9 | 1 | 7 |
| 1 | 4 | 9 | 8 | 2 | 3 | 5 | 7 | 6 |
| 6 | 3 | 5 | 7 | 1 | 4 | 8 | 2 | 9 |
| 7 | 2 | 8 | 6 | 9 | 5 | 1 | 3 | 4 |
| 2 | 1 | 3 | 9 | 8 | 7 | 6 | 4 | 5 |
| 8 | 5 | 4 | 3 | 6 | 1 | 7 | 9 | 2 |
| 9 | 6 | 7 | 4 | 5 | 2 | 3 | 8 | 1 |

# #38

| | | | | | | | | |
|---|---|---|---|---|---|---|---|---|
| 5 | 6 | 1 | 7 | 2 | 4 | 9 | 3 | 8 |
| 9 | 3 | 4 | 8 | 1 | 5 | 6 | 2 | 7 |
| 7 | 2 | 8 | 6 | 9 | 3 | 1 | 4 | 5 |
| 8 | 5 | 2 | 1 | 6 | 9 | 3 | 7 | 4 |
| 3 | 9 | 6 | 5 | 4 | 7 | 2 | 8 | 1 |
| 1 | 4 | 7 | 2 | 3 | 8 | 5 | 9 | 6 |
| 4 | 1 | 5 | 9 | 7 | 2 | 8 | 6 | 3 |
| 2 | 8 | 3 | 4 | 5 | 6 | 7 | 1 | 9 |
| 6 | 7 | 9 | 3 | 8 | 1 | 4 | 5 | 2 |

# #39

| | | | | | | | | |
|---|---|---|---|---|---|---|---|---|
| 3 | 5 | 4 | 2 | 7 | 6 | 8 | 9 | 1 |
| 8 | 6 | 1 | 4 | 3 | 9 | 5 | 7 | 2 |
| 9 | 7 | 2 | 1 | 5 | 8 | 4 | 6 | 3 |
| 5 | 4 | 3 | 9 | 6 | 2 | 7 | 1 | 8 |
| 2 | 1 | 6 | 7 | 8 | 5 | 9 | 3 | 4 |
| 7 | 8 | 9 | 3 | 1 | 4 | 2 | 5 | 6 |
| 6 | 3 | 8 | 5 | 4 | 7 | 1 | 2 | 9 |
| 4 | 9 | 5 | 6 | 2 | 1 | 3 | 8 | 7 |
| 1 | 2 | 7 | 8 | 9 | 3 | 6 | 4 | 5 |

# #40

| | | | | | | | | |
|---|---|---|---|---|---|---|---|---|
| 7 | 2 | 4 | 1 | 8 | 6 | 5 | 3 | 9 |
| 5 | 6 | 1 | 9 | 3 | 4 | 8 | 7 | 2 |
| 9 | 3 | 8 | 5 | 2 | 7 | 6 | 4 | 1 |
| 8 | 4 | 2 | 6 | 1 | 5 | 3 | 9 | 7 |
| 3 | 7 | 5 | 8 | 4 | 9 | 2 | 1 | 6 |
| 6 | 1 | 9 | 3 | 7 | 2 | 4 | 5 | 8 |
| 1 | 5 | 3 | 2 | 9 | 8 | 7 | 6 | 4 |
| 4 | 8 | 6 | 7 | 5 | 1 | 9 | 2 | 3 |
| 2 | 9 | 7 | 4 | 6 | 3 | 1 | 8 | 5 |

# #41

| 9 | 8 | 1 | 5 | 3 | 6 | 2 | 7 | 4 |
|---|---|---|---|---|---|---|---|---|
| 6 | 3 | 7 | 4 | 8 | 2 | 5 | 1 | 9 |
| 5 | 4 | 2 | 7 | 1 | 9 | 6 | 8 | 3 |
| 8 | 2 | 9 | 6 | 4 | 1 | 3 | 5 | 7 |
| 3 | 7 | 6 | 9 | 2 | 5 | 1 | 4 | 8 |
| 4 | 1 | 5 | 3 | 7 | 8 | 9 | 6 | 2 |
| 1 | 5 | 8 | 2 | 9 | 7 | 4 | 3 | 6 |
| 7 | 9 | 4 | 1 | 6 | 3 | 8 | 2 | 5 |
| 2 | 6 | 3 | 8 | 5 | 4 | 7 | 9 | 1 |

# #42

| 9 | 4 | 6 | 8 | 7 | 2 | 3 | 1 | 5 |
|---|---|---|---|---|---|---|---|---|
| 2 | 5 | 3 | 6 | 4 | 1 | 7 | 9 | 8 |
| 7 | 8 | 1 | 3 | 9 | 5 | 6 | 2 | 4 |
| 3 | 7 | 4 | 1 | 8 | 9 | 2 | 5 | 6 |
| 8 | 1 | 5 | 2 | 6 | 7 | 9 | 4 | 3 |
| 6 | 9 | 2 | 4 | 5 | 3 | 1 | 8 | 7 |
| 5 | 2 | 9 | 7 | 3 | 4 | 8 | 6 | 1 |
| 1 | 3 | 8 | 5 | 2 | 6 | 4 | 7 | 9 |
| 4 | 6 | 7 | 9 | 1 | 8 | 5 | 3 | 2 |

# #43

| 8 | 9 | 6 | 4 | 1 | 5 | 2 | 7 | 3 |
|---|---|---|---|---|---|---|---|---|
| 7 | 2 | 5 | 3 | 6 | 9 | 1 | 4 | 8 |
| 4 | 3 | 1 | 8 | 2 | 7 | 9 | 6 | 5 |
| 9 | 1 | 8 | 7 | 5 | 2 | 6 | 3 | 4 |
| 5 | 4 | 7 | 6 | 9 | 3 | 8 | 2 | 1 |
| 3 | 6 | 2 | 1 | 4 | 8 | 7 | 5 | 9 |
| 2 | 7 | 4 | 9 | 3 | 1 | 5 | 8 | 6 |
| 6 | 8 | 9 | 5 | 7 | 4 | 3 | 1 | 2 |
| 1 | 5 | 3 | 2 | 8 | 6 | 4 | 9 | 7 |

# #44

| 3 | 6 | 2 | 9 | 5 | 7 | 1 | 8 | 4 |
|---|---|---|---|---|---|---|---|---|
| 1 | 8 | 7 | 6 | 4 | 3 | 2 | 5 | 9 |
| 4 | 5 | 9 | 8 | 1 | 2 | 7 | 3 | 6 |
| 7 | 4 | 6 | 5 | 9 | 8 | 3 | 1 | 2 |
| 8 | 1 | 3 | 4 | 2 | 6 | 9 | 7 | 5 |
| 2 | 9 | 5 | 7 | 3 | 1 | 4 | 6 | 8 |
| 6 | 7 | 4 | 1 | 8 | 9 | 5 | 2 | 3 |
| 9 | 2 | 1 | 3 | 6 | 5 | 8 | 4 | 7 |
| 5 | 3 | 8 | 2 | 7 | 4 | 6 | 9 | 1 |

## #45

| | | | | | | | | |
|---|---|---|---|---|---|---|---|---|
| 3 | 7 | 9 | 6 | 4 | 1 | 8 | 5 | 2 |
| 4 | 5 | 1 | 3 | 2 | 8 | 6 | 7 | 9 |
| 6 | 8 | 2 | 5 | 7 | 9 | 3 | 4 | 1 |
| 7 | 3 | 5 | 1 | 9 | 6 | 2 | 8 | 4 |
| 2 | 6 | 8 | 4 | 3 | 7 | 1 | 9 | 5 |
| 9 | 1 | 4 | 8 | 5 | 2 | 7 | 3 | 6 |
| 1 | 2 | 3 | 9 | 8 | 4 | 5 | 6 | 7 |
| 5 | 4 | 7 | 2 | 6 | 3 | 9 | 1 | 8 |
| 8 | 9 | 6 | 7 | 1 | 5 | 4 | 2 | 3 |

## #46

| | | | | | | | | |
|---|---|---|---|---|---|---|---|---|
| 2 | 7 | 4 | 3 | 1 | 5 | 8 | 9 | 6 |
| 9 | 1 | 3 | 2 | 6 | 8 | 7 | 4 | 5 |
| 6 | 5 | 8 | 4 | 9 | 7 | 1 | 2 | 3 |
| 5 | 3 | 7 | 1 | 4 | 9 | 6 | 8 | 2 |
| 8 | 9 | 2 | 6 | 7 | 3 | 4 | 5 | 1 |
| 4 | 6 | 1 | 8 | 5 | 2 | 9 | 3 | 7 |
| 7 | 8 | 5 | 9 | 2 | 1 | 3 | 6 | 4 |
| 3 | 2 | 6 | 7 | 8 | 4 | 5 | 1 | 9 |
| 1 | 4 | 9 | 5 | 3 | 6 | 2 | 7 | 8 |

## #47

| | | | | | | | | |
|---|---|---|---|---|---|---|---|---|
| 3 | 5 | 4 | 9 | 1 | 6 | 2 | 8 | 7 |
| 1 | 2 | 6 | 3 | 7 | 8 | 9 | 5 | 4 |
| 9 | 8 | 7 | 5 | 4 | 2 | 6 | 3 | 1 |
| 8 | 7 | 9 | 1 | 3 | 4 | 5 | 2 | 6 |
| 2 | 6 | 3 | 7 | 8 | 5 | 1 | 4 | 9 |
| 5 | 4 | 1 | 2 | 6 | 9 | 8 | 7 | 3 |
| 4 | 1 | 5 | 6 | 2 | 3 | 7 | 9 | 8 |
| 6 | 3 | 2 | 8 | 9 | 7 | 4 | 1 | 5 |
| 7 | 9 | 8 | 4 | 5 | 1 | 3 | 6 | 2 |

## #48

| | | | | | | | | |
|---|---|---|---|---|---|---|---|---|
| 3 | 6 | 8 | 5 | 2 | 4 | 7 | 9 | 1 |
| 2 | 4 | 9 | 1 | 8 | 7 | 5 | 6 | 3 |
| 1 | 7 | 5 | 6 | 9 | 3 | 4 | 2 | 8 |
| 5 | 3 | 2 | 4 | 6 | 1 | 8 | 7 | 9 |
| 7 | 8 | 6 | 9 | 3 | 5 | 1 | 4 | 2 |
| 9 | 1 | 4 | 8 | 7 | 2 | 3 | 5 | 6 |
| 8 | 2 | 1 | 7 | 5 | 9 | 6 | 3 | 4 |
| 6 | 9 | 7 | 3 | 4 | 8 | 2 | 1 | 5 |
| 4 | 5 | 3 | 2 | 1 | 6 | 9 | 8 | 7 |

# #49

| 7 | 5 | 1 | 3 | 6 | 8 | 2 | 9 | 4 |
|---|---|---|---|---|---|---|---|---|
| 3 | 6 | 4 | 1 | 9 | 2 | 5 | 8 | 7 |
| 9 | 8 | 2 | 5 | 7 | 4 | 3 | 1 | 6 |
| 2 | 1 | 7 | 6 | 5 | 9 | 8 | 4 | 3 |
| 6 | 9 | 8 | 4 | 3 | 7 | 1 | 5 | 2 |
| 5 | 4 | 3 | 2 | 8 | 1 | 6 | 7 | 9 |
| 1 | 7 | 5 | 9 | 2 | 3 | 4 | 6 | 8 |
| 4 | 3 | 9 | 8 | 1 | 6 | 7 | 2 | 5 |
| 8 | 2 | 6 | 7 | 4 | 5 | 9 | 3 | 1 |

# #50

| 6 | 5 | 9 | 7 | 3 | 8 | 2 | 1 | 4 |
|---|---|---|---|---|---|---|---|---|
| 2 | 4 | 7 | 6 | 1 | 9 | 5 | 3 | 8 |
| 1 | 3 | 8 | 5 | 2 | 4 | 9 | 6 | 7 |
| 8 | 6 | 5 | 9 | 4 | 7 | 3 | 2 | 1 |
| 4 | 7 | 1 | 3 | 6 | 2 | 8 | 5 | 9 |
| 3 | 9 | 2 | 1 | 8 | 5 | 7 | 4 | 6 |
| 9 | 8 | 6 | 2 | 5 | 1 | 4 | 7 | 3 |
| 5 | 1 | 4 | 8 | 7 | 3 | 6 | 9 | 2 |
| 7 | 2 | 3 | 4 | 9 | 6 | 1 | 8 | 5 |

# #51

| 5 | 9 | 3 | 2 | 4 | 8 | 7 | 6 | 1 |
|---|---|---|---|---|---|---|---|---|
| 2 | 8 | 1 | 3 | 6 | 7 | 4 | 9 | 5 |
| 6 | 4 | 7 | 5 | 9 | 1 | 3 | 2 | 8 |
| 8 | 1 | 9 | 6 | 7 | 3 | 5 | 4 | 2 |
| 7 | 6 | 4 | 9 | 5 | 2 | 1 | 8 | 3 |
| 3 | 2 | 5 | 1 | 8 | 4 | 6 | 7 | 9 |
| 9 | 3 | 6 | 4 | 2 | 5 | 8 | 1 | 7 |
| 4 | 5 | 8 | 7 | 1 | 9 | 2 | 3 | 6 |
| 1 | 7 | 2 | 8 | 3 | 6 | 9 | 5 | 4 |

# #52

| 8 | 5 | 7 | 1 | 4 | 9 | 6 | 3 | 2 |
|---|---|---|---|---|---|---|---|---|
| 3 | 1 | 9 | 6 | 2 | 8 | 7 | 4 | 5 |
| 2 | 4 | 6 | 5 | 7 | 3 | 1 | 8 | 9 |
| 7 | 9 | 4 | 2 | 5 | 6 | 8 | 1 | 3 |
| 6 | 3 | 8 | 4 | 9 | 1 | 5 | 2 | 7 |
| 1 | 2 | 5 | 3 | 8 | 7 | 9 | 6 | 4 |
| 4 | 6 | 1 | 9 | 3 | 5 | 2 | 7 | 8 |
| 5 | 7 | 2 | 8 | 6 | 4 | 3 | 9 | 1 |
| 9 | 8 | 3 | 7 | 1 | 2 | 4 | 5 | 6 |

# #53

| | | | | | | | | |
|---|---|---|---|---|---|---|---|---|
| 5 | 7 | 1 | 6 | 2 | 8 | 4 | 3 | 9 |
| 2 | 6 | 4 | 3 | 9 | 5 | 8 | 1 | 7 |
| 3 | 8 | 9 | 4 | 7 | 1 | 6 | 2 | 5 |
| 1 | 5 | 6 | 2 | 8 | 3 | 9 | 7 | 4 |
| 9 | 3 | 8 | 5 | 4 | 7 | 2 | 6 | 1 |
| 4 | 2 | 7 | 1 | 6 | 9 | 5 | 8 | 3 |
| 7 | 9 | 2 | 8 | 3 | 4 | 1 | 5 | 6 |
| 8 | 1 | 3 | 9 | 5 | 6 | 7 | 4 | 2 |
| 6 | 4 | 5 | 7 | 1 | 2 | 3 | 9 | 8 |

# #54

| | | | | | | | | |
|---|---|---|---|---|---|---|---|---|
| 6 | 4 | 5 | 7 | 9 | 2 | 1 | 3 | 8 |
| 7 | 2 | 3 | 8 | 4 | 1 | 9 | 6 | 5 |
| 1 | 8 | 9 | 5 | 3 | 6 | 2 | 7 | 4 |
| 5 | 3 | 4 | 6 | 1 | 8 | 7 | 9 | 2 |
| 2 | 1 | 8 | 9 | 7 | 4 | 6 | 5 | 3 |
| 9 | 7 | 6 | 3 | 2 | 5 | 4 | 8 | 1 |
| 8 | 5 | 1 | 2 | 6 | 7 | 3 | 4 | 9 |
| 3 | 6 | 2 | 4 | 5 | 9 | 8 | 1 | 7 |
| 4 | 9 | 7 | 1 | 8 | 3 | 5 | 2 | 6 |

# #55

| | | | | | | | | |
|---|---|---|---|---|---|---|---|---|
| 8 | 2 | 4 | 7 | 5 | 6 | 1 | 9 | 3 |
| 6 | 9 | 7 | 3 | 1 | 8 | 5 | 2 | 4 |
| 1 | 3 | 5 | 2 | 9 | 4 | 6 | 8 | 7 |
| 7 | 1 | 2 | 9 | 6 | 3 | 8 | 4 | 5 |
| 5 | 8 | 6 | 4 | 2 | 7 | 9 | 3 | 1 |
| 9 | 4 | 3 | 1 | 8 | 5 | 2 | 7 | 6 |
| 4 | 5 | 9 | 8 | 7 | 1 | 3 | 6 | 2 |
| 3 | 6 | 8 | 5 | 4 | 2 | 7 | 1 | 9 |
| 2 | 7 | 1 | 6 | 3 | 9 | 4 | 5 | 8 |

# #56

| | | | | | | | | |
|---|---|---|---|---|---|---|---|---|
| 4 | 8 | 2 | 9 | 1 | 5 | 6 | 3 | 7 |
| 7 | 5 | 3 | 2 | 6 | 8 | 1 | 4 | 9 |
| 6 | 9 | 1 | 7 | 4 | 3 | 5 | 2 | 8 |
| 8 | 4 | 6 | 1 | 9 | 7 | 2 | 5 | 3 |
| 1 | 3 | 5 | 8 | 2 | 6 | 7 | 9 | 4 |
| 9 | 2 | 7 | 5 | 3 | 4 | 8 | 1 | 6 |
| 2 | 1 | 4 | 6 | 7 | 9 | 3 | 8 | 5 |
| 5 | 6 | 9 | 3 | 8 | 2 | 4 | 7 | 1 |
| 3 | 7 | 8 | 4 | 5 | 1 | 9 | 6 | 2 |

# #57

| | | | | | | | | |
|---|---|---|---|---|---|---|---|---|
| 8 | 4 | 7 | 1 | 6 | 2 | 9 | 5 | 3 |
| 9 | 3 | 2 | 8 | 4 | 5 | 6 | 1 | 7 |
| 1 | 6 | 5 | 3 | 7 | 9 | 4 | 8 | 2 |
| 2 | 8 | 3 | 7 | 5 | 4 | 1 | 6 | 9 |
| 7 | 1 | 6 | 9 | 3 | 8 | 2 | 4 | 5 |
| 5 | 9 | 4 | 2 | 1 | 6 | 7 | 3 | 8 |
| 4 | 5 | 9 | 6 | 8 | 7 | 3 | 2 | 1 |
| 3 | 2 | 8 | 4 | 9 | 1 | 5 | 7 | 6 |
| 6 | 7 | 1 | 5 | 2 | 3 | 8 | 9 | 4 |

# #58

| | | | | | | | | |
|---|---|---|---|---|---|---|---|---|
| 9 | 6 | 3 | 7 | 4 | 8 | 2 | 5 | 1 |
| 7 | 2 | 1 | 6 | 5 | 9 | 8 | 4 | 3 |
| 8 | 5 | 4 | 1 | 3 | 2 | 6 | 7 | 9 |
| 3 | 4 | 7 | 8 | 9 | 5 | 1 | 2 | 6 |
| 6 | 8 | 5 | 2 | 1 | 3 | 4 | 9 | 7 |
| 1 | 9 | 2 | 4 | 6 | 7 | 5 | 3 | 8 |
| 4 | 7 | 8 | 3 | 2 | 6 | 9 | 1 | 5 |
| 2 | 3 | 9 | 5 | 8 | 1 | 7 | 6 | 4 |
| 5 | 1 | 6 | 9 | 7 | 4 | 3 | 8 | 2 |

# #59

| | | | | | | | | |
|---|---|---|---|---|---|---|---|---|
| 8 | 2 | 4 | 6 | 1 | 7 | 9 | 5 | 3 |
| 3 | 9 | 7 | 8 | 4 | 5 | 2 | 1 | 6 |
| 1 | 5 | 6 | 9 | 3 | 2 | 8 | 4 | 7 |
| 7 | 4 | 3 | 2 | 5 | 6 | 1 | 8 | 9 |
| 6 | 1 | 2 | 4 | 8 | 9 | 3 | 7 | 5 |
| 5 | 8 | 9 | 1 | 7 | 3 | 6 | 2 | 4 |
| 2 | 7 | 5 | 3 | 6 | 1 | 4 | 9 | 8 |
| 9 | 3 | 8 | 7 | 2 | 4 | 5 | 6 | 1 |
| 4 | 6 | 1 | 5 | 9 | 8 | 7 | 3 | 2 |

# #60

| | | | | | | | | |
|---|---|---|---|---|---|---|---|---|
| 8 | 9 | 1 | 4 | 6 | 3 | 7 | 5 | 2 |
| 3 | 4 | 5 | 7 | 2 | 9 | 1 | 8 | 6 |
| 2 | 6 | 7 | 1 | 5 | 8 | 4 | 3 | 9 |
| 6 | 3 | 2 | 8 | 4 | 1 | 5 | 9 | 7 |
| 1 | 5 | 4 | 2 | 9 | 7 | 3 | 6 | 8 |
| 9 | 7 | 8 | 5 | 3 | 6 | 2 | 4 | 1 |
| 5 | 1 | 9 | 6 | 7 | 4 | 8 | 2 | 3 |
| 7 | 2 | 3 | 9 | 8 | 5 | 6 | 1 | 4 |
| 4 | 8 | 6 | 3 | 1 | 2 | 9 | 7 | 5 |

## #61

| | | | | | | | | |
|---|---|---|---|---|---|---|---|---|
| 2 | 3 | 6 | 5 | 7 | 1 | 4 | 9 | 8 |
| 1 | 8 | 9 | 3 | 4 | 2 | 5 | 6 | 7 |
| 4 | 5 | 7 | 8 | 9 | 6 | 1 | 3 | 2 |
| 7 | 6 | 1 | 2 | 8 | 4 | 3 | 5 | 9 |
| 5 | 9 | 4 | 1 | 3 | 7 | 8 | 2 | 6 |
| 3 | 2 | 8 | 9 | 6 | 5 | 7 | 1 | 4 |
| 6 | 7 | 5 | 4 | 1 | 9 | 2 | 8 | 3 |
| 9 | 1 | 3 | 7 | 2 | 8 | 6 | 4 | 5 |
| 8 | 4 | 2 | 6 | 5 | 3 | 9 | 7 | 1 |

## #62

| | | | | | | | | |
|---|---|---|---|---|---|---|---|---|
| 4 | 1 | 9 | 5 | 2 | 6 | 7 | 3 | 8 |
| 2 | 6 | 3 | 1 | 7 | 8 | 4 | 9 | 5 |
| 8 | 7 | 5 | 4 | 9 | 3 | 1 | 6 | 2 |
| 6 | 5 | 7 | 9 | 3 | 1 | 8 | 2 | 4 |
| 3 | 4 | 2 | 6 | 8 | 7 | 5 | 1 | 9 |
| 1 | 9 | 8 | 2 | 5 | 4 | 6 | 7 | 3 |
| 7 | 3 | 1 | 8 | 4 | 2 | 9 | 5 | 6 |
| 5 | 2 | 4 | 7 | 6 | 9 | 3 | 8 | 1 |
| 9 | 8 | 6 | 3 | 1 | 5 | 2 | 4 | 7 |

## #63

| | | | | | | | | |
|---|---|---|---|---|---|---|---|---|
| 6 | 9 | 1 | 7 | 3 | 8 | 5 | 2 | 4 |
| 5 | 3 | 2 | 4 | 6 | 9 | 7 | 1 | 8 |
| 7 | 4 | 8 | 5 | 1 | 2 | 6 | 3 | 9 |
| 1 | 8 | 7 | 3 | 4 | 5 | 9 | 6 | 2 |
| 3 | 6 | 9 | 8 | 2 | 7 | 4 | 5 | 1 |
| 4 | 2 | 5 | 1 | 9 | 6 | 3 | 8 | 7 |
| 9 | 5 | 3 | 2 | 8 | 4 | 1 | 7 | 6 |
| 2 | 7 | 4 | 6 | 5 | 1 | 8 | 9 | 3 |
| 8 | 1 | 6 | 9 | 7 | 3 | 2 | 4 | 5 |

## #64

| | | | | | | | | |
|---|---|---|---|---|---|---|---|---|
| 1 | 4 | 8 | 2 | 5 | 7 | 3 | 6 | 9 |
| 7 | 9 | 6 | 8 | 3 | 4 | 1 | 5 | 2 |
| 5 | 3 | 2 | 6 | 9 | 1 | 7 | 4 | 8 |
| 6 | 2 | 7 | 4 | 8 | 5 | 9 | 1 | 3 |
| 4 | 1 | 5 | 9 | 7 | 3 | 2 | 8 | 6 |
| 9 | 8 | 3 | 1 | 2 | 6 | 5 | 7 | 4 |
| 8 | 7 | 9 | 5 | 6 | 2 | 4 | 3 | 1 |
| 3 | 6 | 1 | 7 | 4 | 9 | 8 | 2 | 5 |
| 2 | 5 | 4 | 3 | 1 | 8 | 6 | 9 | 7 |

# #65

| 7 | 2 | 9 | 5 | 8 | 6 | 1 | 4 | 3 |
|---|---|---|---|---|---|---|---|---|
| 5 | 6 | 1 | 3 | 9 | 4 | 2 | 8 | 7 |
| 8 | 4 | 3 | 7 | 2 | 1 | 6 | 9 | 5 |
| 3 | 9 | 7 | 4 | 1 | 8 | 5 | 6 | 2 |
| 4 | 5 | 6 | 2 | 7 | 3 | 9 | 1 | 8 |
| 1 | 8 | 2 | 6 | 5 | 9 | 7 | 3 | 4 |
| 6 | 3 | 5 | 9 | 4 | 7 | 8 | 2 | 1 |
| 2 | 1 | 4 | 8 | 6 | 5 | 3 | 7 | 9 |
| 9 | 7 | 8 | 1 | 3 | 2 | 4 | 5 | 6 |

# #66

| 8 | 5 | 1 | 9 | 7 | 2 | 6 | 3 | 4 |
|---|---|---|---|---|---|---|---|---|
| 3 | 2 | 4 | 8 | 5 | 6 | 1 | 7 | 9 |
| 9 | 7 | 6 | 4 | 3 | 1 | 8 | 2 | 5 |
| 2 | 9 | 7 | 3 | 6 | 4 | 5 | 8 | 1 |
| 6 | 1 | 3 | 5 | 2 | 8 | 9 | 4 | 7 |
| 4 | 8 | 5 | 1 | 9 | 7 | 3 | 6 | 2 |
| 7 | 3 | 2 | 6 | 1 | 5 | 4 | 9 | 8 |
| 1 | 4 | 9 | 2 | 8 | 3 | 7 | 5 | 6 |
| 5 | 6 | 8 | 7 | 4 | 9 | 2 | 1 | 3 |

# #67

| 7 | 1 | 3 | 6 | 5 | 8 | 4 | 2 | 9 |
|---|---|---|---|---|---|---|---|---|
| 8 | 4 | 5 | 7 | 2 | 9 | 6 | 3 | 1 |
| 6 | 9 | 2 | 4 | 3 | 1 | 7 | 8 | 5 |
| 9 | 6 | 7 | 3 | 4 | 2 | 5 | 1 | 8 |
| 1 | 5 | 4 | 9 | 8 | 7 | 3 | 6 | 2 |
| 3 | 2 | 8 | 1 | 6 | 5 | 9 | 4 | 7 |
| 2 | 3 | 1 | 5 | 9 | 6 | 8 | 7 | 4 |
| 5 | 7 | 6 | 8 | 1 | 4 | 2 | 9 | 3 |
| 4 | 8 | 9 | 2 | 7 | 3 | 1 | 5 | 6 |

# #68

| 9 | 5 | 2 | 4 | 8 | 1 | 6 | 7 | 3 |
|---|---|---|---|---|---|---|---|---|
| 7 | 6 | 3 | 2 | 5 | 9 | 8 | 1 | 4 |
| 1 | 8 | 4 | 7 | 3 | 6 | 5 | 9 | 2 |
| 3 | 4 | 9 | 6 | 7 | 5 | 1 | 2 | 8 |
| 2 | 7 | 6 | 1 | 4 | 8 | 9 | 3 | 5 |
| 5 | 1 | 8 | 9 | 2 | 3 | 7 | 4 | 6 |
| 8 | 2 | 1 | 5 | 9 | 4 | 3 | 6 | 7 |
| 4 | 9 | 5 | 3 | 6 | 7 | 2 | 8 | 1 |
| 6 | 3 | 7 | 8 | 1 | 2 | 4 | 5 | 9 |

# #69

| | | | | | | | | |
|---|---|---|---|---|---|---|---|---|
| 3 | 1 | 5 | 2 | 6 | 7 | 4 | 9 | 8 |
| 2 | 7 | 4 | 9 | 8 | 3 | 1 | 5 | 6 |
| 9 | 8 | 6 | 5 | 4 | 1 | 2 | 3 | 7 |
| 8 | 4 | 2 | 3 | 1 | 5 | 7 | 6 | 9 |
| 7 | 6 | 9 | 4 | 2 | 8 | 3 | 1 | 5 |
| 1 | 5 | 3 | 6 | 7 | 9 | 8 | 2 | 4 |
| 4 | 2 | 8 | 1 | 5 | 6 | 9 | 7 | 3 |
| 6 | 3 | 7 | 8 | 9 | 2 | 5 | 4 | 1 |
| 5 | 9 | 1 | 7 | 3 | 4 | 6 | 8 | 2 |

# #70

| | | | | | | | | |
|---|---|---|---|---|---|---|---|---|
| 6 | 7 | 3 | 4 | 5 | 1 | 9 | 2 | 8 |
| 5 | 8 | 4 | 7 | 9 | 2 | 1 | 6 | 3 |
| 9 | 1 | 2 | 3 | 8 | 6 | 4 | 7 | 5 |
| 1 | 3 | 6 | 9 | 4 | 7 | 8 | 5 | 2 |
| 4 | 9 | 8 | 2 | 3 | 5 | 6 | 1 | 7 |
| 7 | 2 | 5 | 1 | 6 | 8 | 3 | 9 | 4 |
| 8 | 4 | 7 | 5 | 1 | 9 | 2 | 3 | 6 |
| 3 | 5 | 1 | 6 | 2 | 4 | 7 | 8 | 9 |
| 2 | 6 | 9 | 8 | 7 | 3 | 5 | 4 | 1 |

# #71

| | | | | | | | | |
|---|---|---|---|---|---|---|---|---|
| 4 | 6 | 2 | 9 | 7 | 5 | 3 | 8 | 1 |
| 9 | 8 | 7 | 6 | 3 | 1 | 2 | 5 | 4 |
| 5 | 1 | 3 | 2 | 4 | 8 | 6 | 9 | 7 |
| 2 | 7 | 8 | 1 | 5 | 6 | 4 | 3 | 9 |
| 3 | 9 | 6 | 8 | 2 | 4 | 7 | 1 | 5 |
| 1 | 5 | 4 | 3 | 9 | 7 | 8 | 2 | 6 |
| 7 | 3 | 9 | 4 | 1 | 2 | 5 | 6 | 8 |
| 6 | 4 | 1 | 5 | 8 | 3 | 9 | 7 | 2 |
| 8 | 2 | 5 | 7 | 6 | 9 | 1 | 4 | 3 |

# #72

| | | | | | | | | |
|---|---|---|---|---|---|---|---|---|
| 8 | 2 | 5 | 9 | 6 | 7 | 1 | 4 | 3 |
| 6 | 9 | 4 | 1 | 3 | 2 | 7 | 5 | 8 |
| 3 | 7 | 1 | 4 | 5 | 8 | 2 | 9 | 6 |
| 1 | 3 | 9 | 8 | 7 | 6 | 5 | 2 | 4 |
| 5 | 8 | 2 | 3 | 4 | 9 | 6 | 7 | 1 |
| 4 | 6 | 7 | 2 | 1 | 5 | 3 | 8 | 9 |
| 2 | 1 | 6 | 7 | 8 | 4 | 9 | 3 | 5 |
| 9 | 5 | 8 | 6 | 2 | 3 | 4 | 1 | 7 |
| 7 | 4 | 3 | 5 | 9 | 1 | 8 | 6 | 2 |

# #73

| 5 | 4 | 7 | 6 | 9 | 2 | 1 | 8 | 3 |
|---|---|---|---|---|---|---|---|---|
| 3 | 9 | 2 | 5 | 8 | 1 | 4 | 6 | 7 |
| 1 | 8 | 6 | 3 | 4 | 7 | 2 | 5 | 9 |
| 6 | 5 | 1 | 4 | 3 | 9 | 7 | 2 | 8 |
| 9 | 7 | 8 | 2 | 6 | 5 | 3 | 4 | 1 |
| 2 | 3 | 4 | 1 | 7 | 8 | 5 | 9 | 6 |
| 4 | 6 | 5 | 9 | 1 | 3 | 8 | 7 | 2 |
| 7 | 2 | 3 | 8 | 5 | 6 | 9 | 1 | 4 |
| 8 | 1 | 9 | 7 | 2 | 4 | 6 | 3 | 5 |

# #74

| 5 | 3 | 1 | 8 | 2 | 4 | 6 | 9 | 7 |
|---|---|---|---|---|---|---|---|---|
| 9 | 7 | 2 | 1 | 6 | 3 | 4 | 5 | 8 |
| 6 | 8 | 4 | 5 | 7 | 9 | 3 | 2 | 1 |
| 8 | 5 | 9 | 4 | 1 | 6 | 2 | 7 | 3 |
| 7 | 1 | 6 | 3 | 9 | 2 | 8 | 4 | 5 |
| 2 | 4 | 3 | 7 | 5 | 8 | 9 | 1 | 6 |
| 3 | 6 | 7 | 9 | 4 | 1 | 5 | 8 | 2 |
| 1 | 9 | 8 | 2 | 3 | 5 | 7 | 6 | 4 |
| 4 | 2 | 5 | 6 | 8 | 7 | 1 | 3 | 9 |

# #75

| 2 | 7 | 4 | 3 | 5 | 9 | 1 | 6 | 8 |
|---|---|---|---|---|---|---|---|---|
| 9 | 1 | 8 | 2 | 4 | 6 | 7 | 3 | 5 |
| 3 | 5 | 6 | 7 | 8 | 1 | 9 | 2 | 4 |
| 6 | 8 | 3 | 4 | 7 | 5 | 2 | 9 | 1 |
| 4 | 2 | 1 | 6 | 9 | 8 | 5 | 7 | 3 |
| 5 | 9 | 7 | 1 | 3 | 2 | 8 | 4 | 6 |
| 8 | 4 | 2 | 5 | 6 | 7 | 3 | 1 | 9 |
| 1 | 3 | 9 | 8 | 2 | 4 | 6 | 5 | 7 |
| 7 | 6 | 5 | 9 | 1 | 3 | 4 | 8 | 2 |

# #76

| 7 | 3 | 9 | 8 | 4 | 2 | 1 | 5 | 6 |
|---|---|---|---|---|---|---|---|---|
| 6 | 8 | 4 | 1 | 5 | 7 | 3 | 9 | 2 |
| 2 | 5 | 1 | 6 | 9 | 3 | 4 | 7 | 8 |
| 1 | 2 | 7 | 3 | 8 | 4 | 9 | 6 | 5 |
| 4 | 6 | 5 | 2 | 7 | 9 | 8 | 1 | 3 |
| 8 | 9 | 3 | 5 | 6 | 1 | 2 | 4 | 7 |
| 5 | 7 | 2 | 4 | 1 | 8 | 6 | 3 | 9 |
| 3 | 1 | 6 | 9 | 2 | 5 | 7 | 8 | 4 |
| 9 | 4 | 8 | 7 | 3 | 6 | 5 | 2 | 1 |

## #77

| | | | | | | | | |
|---|---|---|---|---|---|---|---|---|
| 6 | 1 | 4 | 2 | 7 | 8 | 5 | 9 | 3 |
| 8 | 2 | 3 | 9 | 5 | 4 | 6 | 1 | 7 |
| 5 | 7 | 9 | 6 | 1 | 3 | 4 | 8 | 2 |
| 3 | 9 | 8 | 4 | 6 | 7 | 2 | 5 | 1 |
| 2 | 5 | 6 | 3 | 8 | 1 | 7 | 4 | 9 |
| 1 | 4 | 7 | 5 | 2 | 9 | 8 | 3 | 6 |
| 9 | 8 | 2 | 1 | 4 | 6 | 3 | 7 | 5 |
| 4 | 3 | 5 | 7 | 9 | 2 | 1 | 6 | 8 |
| 7 | 6 | 1 | 8 | 3 | 5 | 9 | 2 | 4 |

## #78

| | | | | | | | | |
|---|---|---|---|---|---|---|---|---|
| 1 | 3 | 7 | 5 | 9 | 4 | 8 | 2 | 6 |
| 4 | 9 | 8 | 2 | 6 | 3 | 5 | 7 | 1 |
| 5 | 6 | 2 | 8 | 1 | 7 | 9 | 4 | 3 |
| 8 | 4 | 5 | 9 | 3 | 1 | 2 | 6 | 7 |
| 2 | 1 | 9 | 7 | 8 | 6 | 3 | 5 | 4 |
| 3 | 7 | 6 | 4 | 2 | 5 | 1 | 8 | 9 |
| 7 | 8 | 4 | 1 | 5 | 9 | 6 | 3 | 2 |
| 6 | 5 | 1 | 3 | 7 | 2 | 4 | 9 | 8 |
| 9 | 2 | 3 | 6 | 4 | 8 | 7 | 1 | 5 |

## #79

| | | | | | | | | |
|---|---|---|---|---|---|---|---|---|
| 9 | 3 | 2 | 7 | 4 | 1 | 5 | 8 | 6 |
| 8 | 7 | 1 | 6 | 9 | 5 | 3 | 4 | 2 |
| 6 | 4 | 5 | 2 | 3 | 8 | 9 | 7 | 1 |
| 4 | 5 | 3 | 8 | 6 | 2 | 7 | 1 | 9 |
| 7 | 6 | 8 | 4 | 1 | 9 | 2 | 5 | 3 |
| 1 | 2 | 9 | 3 | 5 | 7 | 8 | 6 | 4 |
| 5 | 9 | 7 | 1 | 2 | 4 | 6 | 3 | 8 |
| 3 | 8 | 4 | 9 | 7 | 6 | 1 | 2 | 5 |
| 2 | 1 | 6 | 5 | 8 | 3 | 4 | 9 | 7 |

## #80

| | | | | | | | | |
|---|---|---|---|---|---|---|---|---|
| 3 | 4 | 1 | 6 | 5 | 2 | 8 | 7 | 9 |
| 6 | 5 | 7 | 1 | 8 | 9 | 2 | 3 | 4 |
| 8 | 2 | 9 | 4 | 3 | 7 | 6 | 5 | 1 |
| 4 | 1 | 3 | 2 | 7 | 8 | 9 | 6 | 5 |
| 9 | 8 | 6 | 3 | 1 | 5 | 4 | 2 | 7 |
| 5 | 7 | 2 | 9 | 4 | 6 | 3 | 1 | 8 |
| 1 | 9 | 8 | 5 | 2 | 3 | 7 | 4 | 6 |
| 2 | 6 | 4 | 7 | 9 | 1 | 5 | 8 | 3 |
| 7 | 3 | 5 | 8 | 6 | 4 | 1 | 9 | 2 |

# #81

| | | | | | | | | |
|---|---|---|---|---|---|---|---|---|
| 7 | 6 | 4 | 8 | 5 | 1 | 3 | 2 | 9 |
| 1 | 8 | 3 | 9 | 6 | 2 | 7 | 4 | 5 |
| 5 | 2 | 9 | 4 | 3 | 7 | 6 | 1 | 8 |
| 3 | 9 | 7 | 6 | 4 | 5 | 1 | 8 | 2 |
| 2 | 4 | 6 | 1 | 8 | 3 | 9 | 5 | 7 |
| 8 | 5 | 1 | 2 | 7 | 9 | 4 | 6 | 3 |
| 9 | 3 | 8 | 5 | 1 | 4 | 2 | 7 | 6 |
| 6 | 1 | 2 | 7 | 9 | 8 | 5 | 3 | 4 |
| 4 | 7 | 5 | 3 | 2 | 6 | 8 | 9 | 1 |

# #82

| | | | | | | | | |
|---|---|---|---|---|---|---|---|---|
| 3 | 7 | 4 | 2 | 6 | 1 | 9 | 5 | 8 |
| 1 | 9 | 8 | 5 | 7 | 4 | 6 | 2 | 3 |
| 5 | 6 | 2 | 8 | 3 | 9 | 7 | 1 | 4 |
| 7 | 1 | 6 | 9 | 2 | 8 | 3 | 4 | 5 |
| 2 | 5 | 3 | 4 | 1 | 7 | 8 | 6 | 9 |
| 4 | 8 | 9 | 3 | 5 | 6 | 1 | 7 | 2 |
| 6 | 3 | 5 | 7 | 8 | 2 | 4 | 9 | 1 |
| 8 | 4 | 1 | 6 | 9 | 5 | 2 | 3 | 7 |
| 9 | 2 | 7 | 1 | 4 | 3 | 5 | 8 | 6 |

# #83

| | | | | | | | | |
|---|---|---|---|---|---|---|---|---|
| 6 | 8 | 1 | 7 | 5 | 3 | 4 | 9 | 2 |
| 4 | 3 | 9 | 1 | 2 | 6 | 8 | 7 | 5 |
| 2 | 5 | 7 | 4 | 9 | 8 | 1 | 3 | 6 |
| 5 | 4 | 8 | 9 | 1 | 2 | 3 | 6 | 7 |
| 9 | 2 | 6 | 3 | 8 | 7 | 5 | 1 | 4 |
| 1 | 7 | 3 | 6 | 4 | 5 | 2 | 8 | 9 |
| 8 | 6 | 2 | 5 | 7 | 1 | 9 | 4 | 3 |
| 3 | 9 | 5 | 8 | 6 | 4 | 7 | 2 | 1 |
| 7 | 1 | 4 | 2 | 3 | 9 | 6 | 5 | 8 |

# #84

| | | | | | | | | |
|---|---|---|---|---|---|---|---|---|
| 2 | 9 | 3 | 5 | 1 | 8 | 4 | 6 | 7 |
| 1 | 4 | 7 | 2 | 9 | 6 | 3 | 5 | 8 |
| 6 | 8 | 5 | 7 | 4 | 3 | 9 | 2 | 1 |
| 3 | 6 | 2 | 9 | 8 | 7 | 5 | 1 | 4 |
| 7 | 5 | 4 | 3 | 2 | 1 | 6 | 8 | 9 |
| 8 | 1 | 9 | 4 | 6 | 5 | 2 | 7 | 3 |
| 5 | 3 | 6 | 8 | 7 | 4 | 1 | 9 | 2 |
| 4 | 2 | 8 | 1 | 5 | 9 | 7 | 3 | 6 |
| 9 | 7 | 1 | 6 | 3 | 2 | 8 | 4 | 5 |

# #85

| | | | | | | | | |
|---|---|---|---|---|---|---|---|---|
| 3 | 1 | 6 | 4 | 8 | 2 | 9 | 7 | 5 |
| 4 | 9 | 7 | 1 | 6 | 5 | 8 | 2 | 3 |
| 8 | 5 | 2 | 3 | 9 | 7 | 6 | 1 | 4 |
| 2 | 7 | 1 | 8 | 4 | 9 | 5 | 3 | 6 |
| 6 | 8 | 4 | 7 | 5 | 3 | 1 | 9 | 2 |
| 5 | 3 | 9 | 6 | 2 | 1 | 7 | 4 | 8 |
| 7 | 2 | 3 | 5 | 1 | 8 | 4 | 6 | 9 |
| 1 | 4 | 5 | 9 | 3 | 6 | 2 | 8 | 7 |
| 9 | 6 | 8 | 2 | 7 | 4 | 3 | 5 | 1 |

# #86

| | | | | | | | | |
|---|---|---|---|---|---|---|---|---|
| 1 | 2 | 8 | 9 | 6 | 4 | 7 | 5 | 3 |
| 6 | 4 | 7 | 3 | 5 | 1 | 8 | 2 | 9 |
| 5 | 9 | 3 | 7 | 2 | 8 | 4 | 6 | 1 |
| 2 | 7 | 9 | 5 | 1 | 6 | 3 | 4 | 8 |
| 4 | 1 | 5 | 8 | 9 | 3 | 6 | 7 | 2 |
| 3 | 8 | 6 | 4 | 7 | 2 | 1 | 9 | 5 |
| 7 | 5 | 4 | 1 | 8 | 9 | 2 | 3 | 6 |
| 9 | 6 | 1 | 2 | 3 | 7 | 5 | 8 | 4 |
| 8 | 3 | 2 | 6 | 4 | 5 | 9 | 1 | 7 |

# #87

| | | | | | | | | |
|---|---|---|---|---|---|---|---|---|
| 6 | 8 | 7 | 1 | 5 | 9 | 2 | 3 | 4 |
| 9 | 4 | 1 | 3 | 6 | 2 | 5 | 7 | 8 |
| 5 | 2 | 3 | 8 | 7 | 4 | 9 | 1 | 6 |
| 2 | 7 | 5 | 6 | 1 | 3 | 4 | 8 | 9 |
| 8 | 1 | 6 | 4 | 9 | 7 | 3 | 5 | 2 |
| 3 | 9 | 4 | 2 | 8 | 5 | 7 | 6 | 1 |
| 4 | 6 | 2 | 7 | 3 | 1 | 8 | 9 | 5 |
| 1 | 3 | 9 | 5 | 2 | 8 | 6 | 4 | 7 |
| 7 | 5 | 8 | 9 | 4 | 6 | 1 | 2 | 3 |

# #88

| | | | | | | | | |
|---|---|---|---|---|---|---|---|---|
| 5 | 4 | 7 | 9 | 2 | 8 | 3 | 1 | 6 |
| 3 | 1 | 2 | 7 | 4 | 6 | 9 | 5 | 8 |
| 6 | 9 | 8 | 3 | 5 | 1 | 4 | 7 | 2 |
| 4 | 2 | 3 | 8 | 7 | 5 | 6 | 9 | 1 |
| 9 | 5 | 1 | 4 | 6 | 3 | 2 | 8 | 7 |
| 7 | 8 | 6 | 2 | 1 | 9 | 5 | 3 | 4 |
| 2 | 7 | 5 | 1 | 3 | 4 | 8 | 6 | 9 |
| 1 | 6 | 9 | 5 | 8 | 2 | 7 | 4 | 3 |
| 8 | 3 | 4 | 6 | 9 | 7 | 1 | 2 | 5 |

# #89

| 9 | 6 | 2 | 3 | 4 | 8 | 5 | 1 | 7 |
|---|---|---|---|---|---|---|---|---|
| 5 | 8 | 4 | 9 | 7 | 1 | 3 | 2 | 6 |
| 3 | 1 | 7 | 6 | 2 | 5 | 4 | 9 | 8 |
| 8 | 4 | 5 | 7 | 1 | 9 | 6 | 3 | 2 |
| 7 | 2 | 3 | 5 | 8 | 6 | 1 | 4 | 9 |
| 6 | 9 | 1 | 2 | 3 | 4 | 8 | 7 | 5 |
| 4 | 5 | 8 | 1 | 9 | 2 | 7 | 6 | 3 |
| 2 | 7 | 6 | 4 | 5 | 3 | 9 | 8 | 1 |
| 1 | 3 | 9 | 8 | 6 | 7 | 2 | 5 | 4 |

# #90

| 9 | 4 | 3 | 8 | 1 | 7 | 6 | 5 | 2 |
|---|---|---|---|---|---|---|---|---|
| 6 | 1 | 7 | 4 | 2 | 5 | 3 | 8 | 9 |
| 2 | 5 | 8 | 9 | 3 | 6 | 1 | 4 | 7 |
| 7 | 8 | 5 | 3 | 6 | 9 | 2 | 1 | 4 |
| 1 | 2 | 6 | 7 | 5 | 4 | 9 | 3 | 8 |
| 3 | 9 | 4 | 2 | 8 | 1 | 7 | 6 | 5 |
| 5 | 3 | 2 | 1 | 9 | 8 | 4 | 7 | 6 |
| 8 | 7 | 1 | 6 | 4 | 2 | 5 | 9 | 3 |
| 4 | 6 | 9 | 5 | 7 | 3 | 8 | 2 | 1 |

# #91

| 5 | 6 | 2 | 1 | 4 | 7 | 9 | 3 | 8 |
|---|---|---|---|---|---|---|---|---|
| 1 | 9 | 3 | 8 | 5 | 6 | 7 | 2 | 4 |
| 4 | 8 | 7 | 2 | 9 | 3 | 1 | 6 | 5 |
| 8 | 4 | 6 | 3 | 7 | 5 | 2 | 9 | 1 |
| 7 | 2 | 5 | 9 | 1 | 4 | 6 | 8 | 3 |
| 9 | 3 | 1 | 6 | 8 | 2 | 5 | 4 | 7 |
| 6 | 7 | 8 | 4 | 2 | 1 | 3 | 5 | 9 |
| 3 | 5 | 4 | 7 | 6 | 9 | 8 | 1 | 2 |
| 2 | 1 | 9 | 5 | 3 | 8 | 4 | 7 | 6 |

# #92

| 3 | 5 | 9 | 7 | 2 | 4 | 8 | 6 | 1 |
|---|---|---|---|---|---|---|---|---|
| 2 | 7 | 8 | 1 | 3 | 6 | 4 | 9 | 5 |
| 6 | 1 | 4 | 5 | 8 | 9 | 2 | 7 | 3 |
| 5 | 8 | 1 | 9 | 4 | 3 | 6 | 2 | 7 |
| 9 | 6 | 3 | 2 | 7 | 1 | 5 | 4 | 8 |
| 4 | 2 | 7 | 6 | 5 | 8 | 3 | 1 | 9 |
| 8 | 3 | 6 | 4 | 1 | 7 | 9 | 5 | 2 |
| 7 | 9 | 5 | 3 | 6 | 2 | 1 | 8 | 4 |
| 1 | 4 | 2 | 8 | 9 | 5 | 7 | 3 | 6 |

## #93

| | | | | | | | | |
|---|---|---|---|---|---|---|---|---|
| 9 | 1 | 4 | 6 | 7 | 8 | 5 | 2 | 3 |
| 3 | 2 | 6 | 4 | 9 | 5 | 8 | 1 | 7 |
| 8 | 5 | 7 | 3 | 1 | 2 | 6 | 4 | 9 |
| 1 | 9 | 5 | 7 | 2 | 3 | 4 | 8 | 6 |
| 6 | 7 | 3 | 8 | 5 | 4 | 1 | 9 | 2 |
| 2 | 4 | 8 | 1 | 6 | 9 | 3 | 7 | 5 |
| 5 | 3 | 2 | 9 | 8 | 1 | 7 | 6 | 4 |
| 7 | 8 | 9 | 5 | 4 | 6 | 2 | 3 | 1 |
| 4 | 6 | 1 | 2 | 3 | 7 | 9 | 5 | 8 |

## #94

| | | | | | | | | |
|---|---|---|---|---|---|---|---|---|
| 7 | 8 | 2 | 5 | 6 | 9 | 4 | 1 | 3 |
| 9 | 3 | 4 | 2 | 8 | 1 | 7 | 6 | 5 |
| 6 | 1 | 5 | 7 | 4 | 3 | 9 | 8 | 2 |
| 1 | 4 | 8 | 3 | 2 | 6 | 5 | 7 | 9 |
| 2 | 7 | 9 | 8 | 5 | 4 | 1 | 3 | 6 |
| 3 | 5 | 6 | 9 | 1 | 7 | 2 | 4 | 8 |
| 8 | 9 | 7 | 1 | 3 | 2 | 6 | 5 | 4 |
| 5 | 6 | 1 | 4 | 9 | 8 | 3 | 2 | 7 |
| 4 | 2 | 3 | 6 | 7 | 5 | 8 | 9 | 1 |

## #95

| | | | | | | | | |
|---|---|---|---|---|---|---|---|---|
| 3 | 7 | 9 | 4 | 5 | 2 | 8 | 1 | 6 |
| 4 | 8 | 6 | 1 | 9 | 7 | 5 | 2 | 3 |
| 5 | 1 | 2 | 6 | 8 | 3 | 4 | 9 | 7 |
| 1 | 6 | 5 | 9 | 7 | 8 | 3 | 4 | 2 |
| 7 | 3 | 8 | 2 | 4 | 6 | 1 | 5 | 9 |
| 2 | 9 | 4 | 5 | 3 | 1 | 7 | 6 | 8 |
| 8 | 5 | 1 | 3 | 2 | 9 | 6 | 7 | 4 |
| 6 | 2 | 3 | 7 | 1 | 4 | 9 | 8 | 5 |
| 9 | 4 | 7 | 8 | 6 | 5 | 2 | 3 | 1 |

## #96

| | | | | | | | | |
|---|---|---|---|---|---|---|---|---|
| 7 | 5 | 9 | 6 | 2 | 1 | 3 | 4 | 8 |
| 2 | 4 | 8 | 7 | 3 | 9 | 5 | 6 | 1 |
| 3 | 1 | 6 | 8 | 5 | 4 | 7 | 9 | 2 |
| 8 | 7 | 5 | 2 | 1 | 6 | 9 | 3 | 4 |
| 1 | 9 | 4 | 5 | 8 | 3 | 2 | 7 | 6 |
| 6 | 2 | 3 | 9 | 4 | 7 | 8 | 1 | 5 |
| 4 | 8 | 1 | 3 | 7 | 2 | 6 | 5 | 9 |
| 9 | 3 | 2 | 1 | 6 | 5 | 4 | 8 | 7 |
| 5 | 6 | 7 | 4 | 9 | 8 | 1 | 2 | 3 |

# #97

| 6 | 3 | 9 | 1 | 4 | 2 | 7 | 5 | 8 |
|---|---|---|---|---|---|---|---|---|
| 7 | 2 | 8 | 5 | 6 | 9 | 1 | 3 | 4 |
| 5 | 4 | 1 | 3 | 7 | 8 | 2 | 9 | 6 |
| 4 | 8 | 7 | 2 | 9 | 3 | 6 | 1 | 5 |
| 2 | 5 | 3 | 6 | 1 | 7 | 4 | 8 | 9 |
| 1 | 9 | 6 | 4 | 8 | 5 | 3 | 2 | 7 |
| 3 | 7 | 2 | 9 | 5 | 4 | 8 | 6 | 1 |
| 8 | 1 | 5 | 7 | 2 | 6 | 9 | 4 | 3 |
| 9 | 6 | 4 | 8 | 3 | 1 | 5 | 7 | 2 |

# #98

| 2 | 8 | 9 | 6 | 4 | 7 | 1 | 3 | 5 |
|---|---|---|---|---|---|---|---|---|
| 4 | 1 | 5 | 2 | 3 | 8 | 9 | 7 | 6 |
| 7 | 3 | 6 | 9 | 1 | 5 | 2 | 8 | 4 |
| 5 | 6 | 8 | 1 | 2 | 3 | 4 | 9 | 7 |
| 9 | 4 | 1 | 5 | 7 | 6 | 8 | 2 | 3 |
| 3 | 2 | 7 | 8 | 9 | 4 | 5 | 6 | 1 |
| 6 | 5 | 2 | 7 | 8 | 1 | 3 | 4 | 9 |
| 1 | 9 | 4 | 3 | 6 | 2 | 7 | 5 | 8 |
| 8 | 7 | 3 | 4 | 5 | 9 | 6 | 1 | 2 |

# #99

| 1 | 4 | 9 | 6 | 3 | 2 | 5 | 8 | 7 |
|---|---|---|---|---|---|---|---|---|
| 2 | 5 | 6 | 4 | 8 | 7 | 9 | 3 | 1 |
| 3 | 7 | 8 | 5 | 9 | 1 | 2 | 4 | 6 |
| 5 | 2 | 3 | 8 | 1 | 6 | 7 | 9 | 4 |
| 4 | 9 | 1 | 7 | 5 | 3 | 8 | 6 | 2 |
| 8 | 6 | 7 | 2 | 4 | 9 | 3 | 1 | 5 |
| 9 | 1 | 5 | 3 | 2 | 4 | 6 | 7 | 8 |
| 7 | 3 | 2 | 1 | 6 | 8 | 4 | 5 | 9 |
| 6 | 8 | 4 | 9 | 7 | 5 | 1 | 2 | 3 |

# #100

| 1 | 7 | 2 | 8 | 6 | 5 | 4 | 3 | 9 |
|---|---|---|---|---|---|---|---|---|
| 9 | 6 | 4 | 3 | 7 | 2 | 1 | 5 | 8 |
| 8 | 5 | 3 | 4 | 1 | 9 | 7 | 6 | 2 |
| 4 | 3 | 9 | 7 | 5 | 1 | 8 | 2 | 6 |
| 7 | 1 | 5 | 6 | 2 | 8 | 9 | 4 | 3 |
| 2 | 8 | 6 | 9 | 4 | 3 | 5 | 7 | 1 |
| 6 | 2 | 1 | 5 | 9 | 7 | 3 | 8 | 4 |
| 5 | 4 | 8 | 1 | 3 | 6 | 2 | 9 | 7 |
| 3 | 9 | 7 | 2 | 8 | 4 | 6 | 1 | 5 |

www.ingramcontent.com/pod-product-compliance
Lightning Source LLC
Chambersburg PA
CBHW081723250726
48657CB00010B/3103

* 9 7 9 8 5 7 2 8 6 4 0 0 7 *